T0255864

The Management of Stuttering
in Adolescence:
A Communication Skills Approach

To
Diana de Grunwald
for her constant help and encouragement
in the preparation of this manuscript
and
her unfailing support
to families and staff
at the Michael Palin Centre.

The Management of Stuttering in Adolescence: A Communication Skills Approach

Lena Rustin, M.Phil., FCSLT, Reg. MCSLT

Manager of Speech and Language Therapy Services,
Camden and Islington Community Health Services (NHS) Trust.
Michael Palin Centre for Stammering Children, London

Frances Cook, M.Sc., Reg. MCSLT

Principal Speech and Language Therapist
Michael Palin Centre for Stammering Children, London

Rob Spence, M.Sc., Reg. MCSLT

Chief Speech and Language Therapist for Community Health Services,
Camden and Islington Community Health Services (NHS) Trust.
Michael Palin Centre for Stammering Children, London

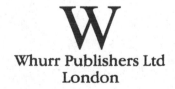

Whurr Publishers Ltd
London

© 1995 Whurr Publishers Ltd

First published 1995 by
Whurr Publishers Ltd
19b Compton Terrace, London N1 2UN, England

Reprinted 1998

All rights reserved. No part of this publication may be reproduced,
stored in a retrieval system, or transmitted in any form or by any
means, electronic, mechanical, photocopying, recording or otherwise,
without the prior permission of Whurr Publishers Limited.

This publication is sold subject to the conditions that it shall not, by
way of trade or otherwise, be lent, resold, hired out, or otherwise
circulated without the publisher's prior consent in any form of
binding or cover other than that in which it is published and without
a similar condition including this condition being imposed upon any
subsequent purchaser.

British Library Cataloguing in Publication Data
A catalogue record for this book is available from the
British Library.

ISBN 1-897635-60-5

Singular no. 1-56593-277-3

Contents

Dedication   ii
Foreword   ix
Preface   x
Acknowledgements   xii

Chapter 1

Introduction   1
The therapeutic relationship   2
The nature of stuttering: an overview   2
The nature of adolescence   6
The adolescent who stutters   8
Summary   14

Chapter 2

The assessment of the adolescent who stutters   15
The interview procedure   16
The diagnostic interview   18
Language assessments   25
The parental interview   26
Further assessments   28
Outcome measures   32

Chapter 3

Planning interventions   37
Physiological factors   38
Cognitive–emotional factors   39
Behavioural factors   39
Environmental factors   39
Four case study presentations   40
Summary   56

Chapter 4

Communication skills approach	**57**
Self-concepts and relationships	57
Components of the communication skills therapy	59

Chapter 5

Intensive group management of adolescents who stutter	**71**
Intensive course procedure	72
Criteria for acceptance on the course	72
Organisation of the course	73
Course assessments	74
Principles of group management	75
Structure of the course	77
Week 2	101

Chapter 6

Environmental influences	**110**
Family involvement	110
The role of the speech and language therapist	111
Child-rearing styles	112
Family interventions	113
Parent-centred sessions	113
Strategies for intervention	117
Intervention within the school setting	122

Chapter 7

Language impairment and the adolescent who stutters	**127**
Claire Topping	
Assessment of language skills	129
Intervention	135
Summary	141

Appendix I	
Initial assessment form	**143**

Appendix II	
Adolescent interview	**144**

Appendix III	
Facts about stuttering	**151**

Appendix IV	
Assessment booklet	**152**

Appendix V
Checklist of social skills   160

Appendix VI
Social communication skills   161

Appendix VII
Measurement of change and outcome   162

Appendix VIII
Measurement of change   163

Appendix IX
The communication skills workbook   167

Appendix X
Examples of self-characterisation   175

Appendix XI
Examples of brainstorm exercises   176

Appendix XII
**Communication, observation, listening, praise and
reinforcement**   177

Appendix XIII
Fear of stuttering; ring of confidence   179

Appendix XIV
Adolescents' view of adolescence   180

Appendix XV
How adolescents think parents' view adolescence   181

Appendix XVI
Parents' view of adolescence   182

Appendix XVII
Family session   183

Appendix XVIII
Review of communication skills course   184

References   **187**

Index   **193**

Foreword

Over the past 15 years, stuttering therapy has started to move away from a narrow focus on fluency toward a broader perspective on the whole person. This book marks a major new step in this progression. Lena Rustin, Frances Cook and Rob Spence have drawn on their rich experiences with young people who stutter to produce this practical book describing an integration of many approaches to help teenagers who stutter.

The core of this therapy combines work on speech fluency with training on social and self-management skills in an intensive group setting. Treatment also brings the family into therapy so that family interactions can be changed to facilitate fluency and enhance communication. This broad-spectrum approach may alleviate some of the problems many have had with teenagers who stutter, such as lack of motivation and poor carryover of results. Moreover, the content of this book is in harmony with the recent trends to integrate therapy with classroom performance. For example, Chapter 7, by Claire Topping, on teenagers whose stuttering is compounded with specific language impairment is rich with ideas and examples for assessment and treatment which are ideal for the school environment.

In addition to the relevant content, this book is written in an accessible and practical manner. The beginning gives us understanding of that baffling condition called adolescence, and renewed hope that we can help these individuals. The middle fully describes assessment and planning of treatment. Then, the remainder is chock-a-block with details of what the authors do in treatment and how they do it. All of this is illustrated with numerous case studies that enable us to appreciate how a carefully planned approach can be adapted to individual clients with their own unique needs.

The reader is now about to begin a delightful educational experience, learning new ways to facilitate behavioural, cognitive, and emotional change in the people they work with and enjoying the insights of three sensible and wise clinicians.

Professor Barry Guitar
University of Vermont

Preface

Adolescents who stutter are viewed by many speech and language therapists as a most difficult client group to treat. This may be attributed to this particular phase of life; to the changing nature of the dysfluency or, perhaps to environmental factors which assume increasing importance within this age group. This book presents the communication skills approach to the management of stuttering in adolescence which has been developed over 20 years of clinical practice.

Chapter 1 describes the central tenets of the approach. Following the introduction, we discuss the importance of the therapeutic relationship, the nature and development of stuttering in adolescence and the adolescent who stutters.

Thus we offer an overview of current research trends and accumulated evidence which define the issues concerning the development of stuttering. The complexity of adolescence, this transitional phase from childhood to adulthood, is then discussed. The 'double trouble' of the adolescent who stutters is then considered with an appraisal of the role of parents, peers and school as factors in management.

Chapter 2 presents the assessment protocol which is fundamental in gaining a comprehensive picture of the adolescent client. The importance of a client-centred approach is emphasised. Adolescent clients frequently have a long and frustrating history of being instructed in what to do by well-meaning adults, including parents, teachers and speech and language therapists, and still have a protracted history of the communication problem. This full assessment gives equal weight to the views and opinions of both the adolescent who stutters and his parents. Thus, a feeling of being in control is engendered and of entering a partnership in the therapeutic process.

Chapter 3 proposes a methodology to assist the clinician in summarising the information that has been obtained in order to formulate an appropriate management plan. Case studies are presented to illustrate the complexity of the possible assessment outcomes. The emphasis here is that the speech problem may not be the first focus in the therapy schedule. For example, it may have been identified that environmental issues will need to be stabilised in the first instance, or that there may be a lack of motivation on the part of the adolescent with the drive for therapy stemming from highly anxious parents.

It is clear that before embarking on any therapy programme, the timing should be right, the package of care appropriate — fully discussed and agreed, and the expectations of therapy examined.

Chapter 4 lays the foundation for the communication skills approach. The components of the therapy programme are described. Throughout, we emphasize that speech modification is only one aspect of therapy and shares equal importance with social skills, problem-solving, relaxation, negotiation and the environmental aspects.

Chapter 5 elaborates the communication skills approach through a detailed description of our 2-week intensive group therapy course. The chapter is structured to demonstrate the overall aims of the daily schedules, with an explanation and rationale for each step. Forms, workbooks and examples are included in the Appendices.

Chapter 6 considers the environmental aspects in the management of the adolescent who stutters. Parental involvement, peer group pressures and aspects of school life are discussed with a variety of management approaches illustrated by case studies.

Finally, Chapter 7, by Claire Topping, offers further guidance for the management of those clients with additional specific language impairment. Assessment procedures and therapy options are proposed. Case studies are again included for illustration.

Acknowledgements

We should like to express our grateful thanks to Jane Fry, Willie Botterill, Elaine Kelman, and Alison Nicholas for their invaluable advice and support throughout the preparation of this text. We also wish to thank Patricia Brown for her contribution to the typing and for the excellence of her 'office skills'.

In addition, we would like to thank Hanna Klein for her helpful suggestions.

Finally, we would like to express our gratitude to Professor Barry Guitar for giving of his time in reading and appraising the manuscript.

Chapter 1
Introduction

Although there have been many advances in our knowledge concerning the complexities of onset and development of stuttering, and despite the publication of many treatment approaches and programmes, speech and language therapists continue to be wary of working with clients who stutter (Cooper and Rustin, 1985). This is particularly the case with the adolescent age group.

The literature concerning onset and development suggests that most stuttering begins in childhood. The latest research indicates that the onset is earlier than previously reported. Yairi (1993) demonstrates a clear tendency for its occurrence under 3 years of age, with females beginning significantly in advance of males. This is attributed to the earlier maturation of the central nervous system in females and lends support to the findings of a strong relationship between onset of stuttering and speech and language development.

The research evidence on spontaneous recovery rates in children varies widely. Andrews et al. (1983) reported recovery rates from 23–80% and Starkweather (1987) stated that 20% and perhaps as many as 50% of children may continue to stutter. Andrews et al. (1983) also noted that the percentage of spontaneous remission decreased from 40%, for those individuals stuttering longer than a year, to 18% spontaneous remission for those stuttering for more than 5 years. It would therefore seem reasonable to infer that adolescents who stutter have been doing so for some time and that there is a rapidly diminishing likelihood of spontaneous recovery in these individuals.

In trying to define the particular problems of the adolescent who stutters, one must not get sidetracked by the research into causation nor the evidence from the research into adult stuttering. The interaction of constitutional, developmental and environmental issues does not need to be addressed in the sense of prevention or possible 'cure', but in the light of how much the stuttering affects the lifestyle, self-image and educational progress of the client, and the functioning of the family as a whole.

In order to design an effective intervention programme it is not only necessary for the clinician to have a sound knowledge of the theoretical issues concerning the nature of stuttering but also to have an understanding of the process of 'adolescence' with its radical and disturbing changes taking place in the transition from childhood to adulthood. The clinician will need to account for both in an individual therapy programme.

The aim of this book is to describe therapy intervention for the adolescent who stutters which accounts for these wide-ranging issues. A particular feature will be to bridge the gap between those children whose parents are an integral part of therapy (Rustin, 1987a; 1987b), and the young adult who is in the process of becoming an independent decision-maker while continuing to be strongly influenced by his family.

The therapeutic relationship

For any therapy programme to be effective it should be credible to both the clinician and client. A sceptical clinician will quickly lose faith in the therapy process, and the adolescent who has had periods of unsuccessful therapy will question the underlying rationale—particularly if aspects challenge his personal beliefs about himself and his stuttering. Both could collude in 'sabotaging' the therapy.

The clinician with a clear understanding of stuttering and its development is better able to select a programme of therapy which is credible, practicable and effective. The client who is given maximum information about the 'state of the art' theories and therapies will be able to make a properly informed decision before embarking on the often painful and difficult process of therapy. Moreover, this would assist in the formation of a partnership between therapist and client with joint responsibility for progress, evaluation and the development of new directions. This sense of shared responsibility is essential with adolescent clients—it precludes the likelihood of over-dependence upon the therapist and allows the adolescent to develop a clearer sense of self determination in overcoming problems.

The nature of stuttering: an overview

This brief overview will identify current thinking in terms of aetiology, onset and development of stuttering, and address the issues of particular relevance to the adolescent who stutters. The aim will be to put theory into the context of therapy.

Most authorities now consider that stuttering is not a homogeneous disorder but 'the problem of many causes' and the 'disorder of many theories'. Van Riper (1982) aptly describes stuttering as 'at least, a complicated, multidimensional jigsaw puzzle, with many pieces still missing'.

It is widely accepted that there is no *single* cause of stuttering, rather a complex interplay between constitutional, developmental, environmental and psychological factors. These categories may be seen in terms of *predisposing* and *precipitating* factors.

Constitutional (predisposing)

Kidd (1984) compares stuttering with asthma, migraine and certain other disorders in terms of being the result of a combination of heredity, the environment and chance factors acting together. Many research studies have indicated that there is a higher incidence of stuttering amongst relatives of people who stutter (Andrews and Harris, 1964; Rustin, 1991). In addition, although there is a preponderance of stuttering amongst males, the relatives of female stutterers are at greater risk (Kidd, 1977; Kidd, Kidd and Records, 1978). Studies of identical twins demonstrate a higher concordance for stuttering than fraternal twins. However, in some identical twin pairs this concordance was not evident, suggesting that environmental influences were coming into play (Howie, 1981). It is unclear what is inherited, but it may be that one or several predisposing factors, interacting with the environment, have to be present for the syndrome of stuttering to be triggered.

Evidence is also available that people who stutter differ from those who do not in terms of linguistic development (Bloodstein, 1987) and sensory motor processing (Peters and Guitar, 1991). They perform less well on tests of linguistic ability at an early age (Bloodstein, 1987) and demonstrate an increase in dysfluencies as language complexity is increased (Bernstein-Ratner and Sih, 1987). It is also reported that dysfluencies occur more frequently at clause boundaries where language is being formulated (Wall, 1977; Kline and Starkweather, 1979). As a group, people who stutter show slightly lower verbal and non-verbal IQ scores (Bloodstein, 1987), and are more likely to have delays in language and in phonological development (Andrews and Harris, 1964; Kline and Starkweather, 1979; Wall, 1980).

Research into neurological factors shows that people who stutter have some differences in cerebral dominance for language and have slower reaction times in voice onset and voice termination tasks (see Peters and Guitar, 1991, for a review). This area of research continues to generate important considerations concerning the fluent utterances of people who stutter. A recent article by Lees (in press) examines recent evidence pertaining to 'subclinical stuttering' as well as the long-term question regarding the heterogeneity of this population.

However, it is clear that these differences do not cause the development of stuttering but it would seem that they may be part of the 'predisposing' aspect of this complex disorder.

Environmental and developmental (precipitating)

These closely interlinked factors may be seen as the determinants responsible for the development or the amelioration of stuttering.

The interplay between physical, cognitive and linguistic development is complex and constantly changing. All aspects impose pressures on an immature neurological system and, although the relationship between these rapidly developing systems and fluency skills is not clear, many authors believe that stuttering may be partly the result of a neurological 'overload'. The rapid physical changes which occur in children from 0–6 years may be competing with the cognitive and linguistic development for the available neurological resources.

The rate of development is dictated by the individual and the environment. If the inherent developmental system is outstretched by social and environmental demands, this may trigger an innate predisposition for stuttering.

The environmental issues include family situation and lifestyle, parental attitudes and philosophies, the child's place within the family and the variable life events that may be relevant.

Starkweather (1987) accounts for both the constitutional and developmental research in his 'Demands and Capacities Model of Fluency Development'. He explains that children's early attempts at conveying ideas may lack fluency, but as they mature they learn to deal with fluency lapses. This growing capacity to talk more easily (language) is paralleled by increasing demands for fluent speech. When the child's capacity for fluency exceeds the demands, the child will talk fluently, but when the child lacks the capacity to meet the demands for fluency, stuttering may develop.

Starkweather (1987) hypothesises that at those moments when the *demands* on fluency are greater than the *capacity*, the child will inevitably try harder to produce speech. This results in tense, uncoordinated speech musculature and with this there could be a growing awareness of a problem, both from the child's and from the parents' perspective. A pattern of struggle, tension and emotional reaction may become habitual and thus stuttering develops.

The notion of a 'capacity for fluency' includes the development of the complex coordination of the vocal tract musculature. The demands for fluency may be seen as both 'internal' and 'external'. The development of language skills, including syntactic, semantic, phonologic and pragmatic knowledge, contribute to the internal demand for fluency. The external demand includes the environmental factors, such as parents, siblings, peers, relatives, and teachers. For example, Starkweather

(1987) suggests that fast parental speech models would naturally be reflected by the child, inadvertently placing a demand for rapid speech on a system which may not be able to cope at that time. Similarly, competition for talking time in a busy household places a demand on the capacity for fluency, as does complex vocabulary and syntax within the speech environment. Starkweather's (1987) model offers an explanation for both the development of fluency and stuttering. In a practical sense, merely examining the complexity of the aetiologies of stuttering may seem less relevant when considering therapy, but the person who stutters and his family should have an understanding of these issues. The greater the client's knowledge about the development of stuttering, the clearer will be his expectations of himself, the therapy process and the therapist.

Onset

Most stuttering begins in childhood without an 'apparent' link to either psychological or organic trauma. Onset is often gradual and interspersed with frequent periods of fluency. Most researchers agree that it may appear from 18 months to 12 years of age, but is most likely between 2–5 years. Onset therefore coincides with a period of rapid language development. As stated above, evidence is growing that many children who stutter have associated speech and language delay.

Prevalence and incidence

The figures vary because of the differing methodologies used in the many studies, with some giving incidence figures as high as 16%. Peters and Guitar (1991) discuss the variables and suggest in their review that the probable incidence of stuttering is about 5% and the prevalence 1%. The difference in these figures may reflect the spontaneous recovery findings.

Sex ratio

Yairi (1983) demonstrated that in 2–3-year-olds the ratio of males to females is 1:1. Bloodstein (1987) puts the ratio at 3:1 in 6–7-year-olds and 5:1 in 12–13-year-olds. Several developmental studies have concluded that the remission of stuttering is much more common in girls than in boys, and there is consequently an increasing preponderance of stuttering in males with age. (Andrews and Harris, 1964; Neaves, 1970; Quinn and Andrews, 1977).

Many authors have described the stages or phases of the development of stuttering. Van Riper (1982) describes the 'core' behaviours of stuttering as involuntary repetitions, prolongations and blocks. Repetitions are mainly characteristic of early childhood stuttering, with prolongations and blocks being more a feature of the developing problem. The 'secondary' characteristics are the result of 'learned reactions' to the core behaviours. He described these characteristics as escape behaviours (facial grimacing, physical movements, etc.) and avoidance behaviours (changing words, postponements, etc.). All are psychologically bound up with the feelings and attitudes towards stuttering of both the individual and the culture.

Bloodstein (1970) in discussing his 'Continuity Hypothesis' of stuttering saw the clinical disorder as a 'more extreme degree of certain forms of normal dysfluency'. He suggested four 'phases' in the developing problem. Phase 1 accounts for the 'normal non-fluencies' of younger children which may persist up to 7 years of age with episodic dysfluencies, no fear or embarrassment, no self-image of being a person who stutters, no avoidances and often no further problems. His Phase 2 depicts the 'more chronic' problem with fewer fluent periods, more predictable patterns, and changes in self-image but no situational avoidance. Phase 3 demonstrates many of the adolescent stutterer's characteristics: difficulties with certain words, anticipation of problems, strategies and devices becoming evident, but still not the elaborately developed symptomatology of the adult chronic problem outlined in his Phase 4.

The controversy is still current between whether stuttering arises out of normal non-fluency or is qualitatively different from the onset. These arguments are important to understand and, in addition, the adolescent and adult who stutter must become aware of the normality and acceptability of common dysfluencies and the part that their own anxiety, awareness, and feeling of panic plays in creating this 'syndrome of stuttering'.

For those children and adolescents whose speech difficulties do not remit, the prospect of the dysfluency developing into a severe and chronic handicap in adult life is a reality.

As stated above, the available evidence on the development of dysfluency consistently points to an increasing risk for the chronic syndrome as the problem persists into adolescence. Therefore, when working with an adolescent client, this high risk of persistent dysfluency in adulthood must be taken into consideration. There is a need therefore for more research into assessment and treatment of the adolescent population in order to understand the specific nature of the adolescent problem and prevent the subsequent development of the complex chronic problem associated with dysfluency in adulthood.

The nature of adolescence

There are number of clear themes of adolescent development and in the following chapter on assessment each of these will be examined separately and then summarised in order to demonstrate the importance of understanding the adolescent as a whole before any therapeutic intervention programme can be instituted. These themes are basic to our understanding of adolescence as being a time of both change and consolidation.

There are major physical transformations which carry with them alterations in body image and, therefore, in the sense of self. There can be little doubt that the physiological developments that occur during this time are amongst the most important events for adolescent adjustment. The process is complex and includes not only changes in the reproductive system and the secondary sexual characteristics, but in the heart and cardiovascular system, the lungs and respiratory system, and in the size and strength of many of the muscle groups of the body.

Intellectual growth makes possible a more complex and sophisticated self-concept, which in turn affects the increasing emotional independence and the approach of fundamental decisions in relation to occupation, personal values, sexual behaviour, friendship choices and the development of social roles.

The study of adolescence has changed perceptibly over the last few years, partly as a result of the social changes that have occurred in Western countries, but more particularly because of recent research which has led to a more realistic view of where 'adolescence' fits into developmental psychology.

The emphasis is changing from the traditional focus on the first five years of life to a broader perspective which encompasses development from birth to early adult life. At one time, psychologists saw early experiences as laying the foundations for later personality development, with the implication of potential irreparable damage which could result from problems at this early stage. The perspective has widened and the adolescent need not be a 'victim of his biography'; there is still, in adolescence, the opportunity for personality growth and development to ensure a healthy approach to adulthood. Adolescence is no longer seen as a static stage, or a number of stages. It is a transitional process of time which results from a variety of pressures both internal and external. These are those physiological changes already cited as well as the environmental pressures from peers, parents, teachers and society. It is the interplay of these demands which contributes to the success or failure of this transitional stage from childhood to adulthood. It is relevant to compare these new pressures with the demands and capacities model of Starkweather (1987), discussed above, in relation to stuttering development. Clearly, the developing capacities and new demands that are being made in this age group will contribute to our understanding of the therapeutic requirements for adolescents who stutter.

'Lifespan Developmental Psychology' is emerging as a useful and practical base from which to understand the transitions of adolescence (Belsky, Lerner and Spannier, 1984). Its assumptions include:

1. The existence of a human ecology: a person develops in the context of the family and within a geographic, historical, social and political setting.
2. Individuals and their families are reciprocal: this suggests that neither the child nor family is a static entity. Each is developing and changing and influencing the other members. The maturing child produces changes within the family but the alterations in family functioning and structure also have effects on the child.
3. Individuals influence their own development: here it is suggested that the young person is an 'active agent' in shaping his own development. This variable must be taken into consideration both in the context of this book, and the therapeutic process when considering the adolescent who stutters.

This approach to developmental psychology sets the stage for our understanding of the process of adolescence and the factors which must be accounted for when considering the particular problems of the adolescent who stutters.

Lerner (1985) considered three ways in which the adolescent interacts with the environment and thereby affects his own development:

1. As a stimulus: eliciting different reactions from the environment.
2. As processor: making sense of the behaviour of others.
3. As agent, shaper and selector: doing things, making choices and influencing events.

Clearly, the speech and language therapist needs to be fully aware of the internal and external demands facing the young adult who stutters, as well as his innate capacities and skills in relation both to speech and social situations. In order to do this a full assessment of the adolescent must include the variables which are present within the family, educational, social, geographical, historical and environmental settings.

The adolescent who stutters

It is widely accepted that the majority of children who grow out of stuttering will do so by adolescence or early adulthood. The research literature has not explained this phenomenon adequately and leaves the clinician questioning the factors which may be responsible for the development of the chronic problem.

One might speculate that remission could be the result of neurological maturation and that the capacity for fluency has achieved an equilibrium with the demands, both in terms of sensory motor processing skills and other possible linguistic factors. Perhaps psychologically the maturing adolescent will be taking more responsibility for his developing self-image and this shift in his locus of control (see p. 12 this chapter) may underpin the recovery. These speculative ideas are underpinned by anecdotal evidence from 'ex-stutterers' who, when asked what they did to overcome the problem, explained '*I decided to take no notice of what others thought of me*', '*I decided to play the game my way*', '*I realised it was up to me and no one else could really help*'.

What then is the problem for the adolescent who continues to stutter? An unresolved neurological problem? A high-level linguistic deficit? Or, the development of the 'stuttering self-image'? It is probably a combination of all these factors. Our experience suggests that many of these clients have rapid rates of speech and often have high-level word retrieval problems. But perhaps the issue of self-concept is the key to the mystery.

Perkins (1992) promotes his theory that stuttering is the result of a 'dominance conflict'. He argues that the need to be assertive is an innate characteristic arising, in evolutionary terms, from the 'survival of the fittest' instinct. He suggests that human interaction is governed hierarchically, with 'dominance' being a fundamental feature—'All men are born equal, but some are more equal than others'. Our communication attempts are influenced by the relative status of the person with whom we are interacting. As long as we are comfortable with our status, no conflict about dominance exists. The dominance conflict arises when a speaker has an innate drive to be assertive (i.e. have control) in a speaking situation but is thwarted both by the other speaker's dominance and his own inability to assert. The conflict is this inability to claim this natural right of being 'assertive'. Perkins (1992) elaborates the argument to address the notion of the pay offs of stuttering. When one is assertive, it is easy to 'control' a conversation. When one is stuttering, the 'pay-off' may be that one becomes able to control the conversation, albeit in a different way.

Thus, a critical factor in Perkins' theory is that the child who does not outgrow the problem has discovered addictive pay-offs which turn stuttering into a powerful tool for dealing with the assertiveness drive. It becomes a safe way of asserting oneself. He describes the pay-offs in terms of parental concern, gaining attention, control of conversations, and the development of fantasies concerning self-image ('giant in chains', '*If only I were fluent, I would be ... rich/powerful/popular*') and that perhaps stuttering may be an effective method of being in control without being openly assertive, aggressive, or angry.

Perkins further suggests that it takes some time before the pay-offs of stuttering become addictive. When they do, people who stutter then build their lives around the image of themselves as stutterers. Speech is seen as the source of power; as a stutterer they are unable to use that power—they are also therefore protected from having to test this theory in the real world.

The critical timing of this development is during adolescence and therefore could perhaps explain the development from stuttering (dysfluency) to stutterer and the adult chronic syndrome.

Social skills

Perkins (1947) commented on the inadequacies of social functioning and social attitudes among children who stutter. Both Prins (1972) and Wingate (1962) concur that over the broad range of measures (self-report, behavioural and observational) children and adolescents who stutter do show more difficulties with social adjustment than children who are fluent. These difficulties include poor interpersonal skills, avoidance of social contact, withdrawal from social interaction and low rates of initiating social contact. The extent to which social and interpersonal difficulties are addressed within contemporary treatment programmes is not always obvious. Rather, treatment schemes have emerged which reflect the most typical form of clinical work, that is, individual sessions of up to 60 minutes on a weekly basis with an implicit focus on individual speech performance, almost regardless of the social context of conversations.

As discussed above, the adolescent has some acute and very particular problems linked to the extensive mental and physical changes taking place at this time: the development of self-awareness and self-doubt; the early experiments with independence and decision-making; concerns about sexuality, both in terms of bodily changes and mental set; increasing demands educationally; changing relationships within the family and within peer group relationships. During this time most adolescents are beginning to accept their strengths and weaknesses, experimenting with decision-making, taking risks and coping with the inevitable failures that occur in pursuing their struggle for independence. Adolescents who stutter may learn to blame their failures on their stuttering, thus avoiding the painful but important experience of having to take personal responsibility for their own actions.

We have noted that many adult clients who stutter have not developed the skills required for normal social interactions. There are well documented difficulties in the transfer and maintenance of fluency which may be linked with deficiencies in adolescent experiences. Indeed, speech and language clinicians are showing an increasing interest in the possible psychological factors which may be contributing to the problem of maintenance of fluency. We would speculate that the person who stutters may have attributed the problems of adolescence to stuttering rather than learning to accept true strengths and weaknesses as they naturally evolve.

The role of parents

As we have discussed, we favour the interactionist model of stuttering development. This suggests a constitutional predisposition to the problem with environmental factors playing a part in precipitating (and conversely in preventing) the emergence and maintenance of the problem. Clearly, although nothing can change the constitutional predisposition, environmental issues can be addressed productively. Virtually all contributors to our understanding of the nature of stuttering have acknowledged the influence of environmental factors and an increasing number do incorporate these issues into their therapy programmes.

Sheehan (1975) and Glasner and Rosenthal (1957) emphasised the child's interpersonal relationships in the family as primary in the development of the problem, whereas even those who have investigated the genetics of stuttering (Kidd, 1984) assume that physiological predispositions and environmental factors interact.

A further argument for involving both parents and others in therapy comes from adults who stutter. Recurring comments demonstrate that in their early years parents would not discuss their stuttering:

- *'I felt isolated, misunderstood and frustrated.'*
- *'Stuttering was a bad thing, something to be ashamed of.'*
- *'I never speak to my parents now about my stutter and they certainly never discussed it with me when I was a child.'*

One can only guess at the internal distress that a child with a stuttering problem must suffer when he is aware that something is wrong, is unable to discuss it and only sees the negative reactions of others to his attempts at communication. After all, what better way is there to draw attention to a problem than by pretending to ignore it? This 'conspiracy of silence' damages trust within the parent–child relationship and contributes to the negative self-image surrounding the stuttering.

The belief that if stuttering was ignored it would go away, was propagated over past years. Until recently speech and language therapy students were taught to offer 'advice' only to parents of children under 7 years—indeed, other professionals still persist with this inappropriate counselling.

The consensus of evidence from national studies in Western countries indicates that the home has more influence on a child's learning than does school (McConkey, 1985). The child's actions are, to a degree, governed by characteristics of the family's system—he may be responding to stresses within the family unit or, indeed, contributing to stressing other members within the family system (Minuchin, 1974). The child who stutters lives within a family and is a member of a social system within which he learns to adapt, and therefore therapy can only be truly effective if account is taken of all aspects of the developing problem. The benefits of involving parents in therapy include: the maintenance of specific skills taught to the child; greater parental awareness and understanding of the child's problem, and the difficulties encountered before, during and after intervention. Parental involvement provides continuity and a prolongation of therapeutic benefits for both the child and themselves.

However, the role of parents changes as their child reaches the nexus between childhood and adulthood. Our aim is to encourage a partnership that will assist in the development of independence, growth of decision-making and ability to negotiate areas of disagreement. Other authority figures (teachers, relatives, etc.) also loom large in the life of the adolescent client. In many cases adolescents are endeavouring to establish their own autonomy in a reasonable way, but in some cases there is a rejection of or rebelliousness towards every person seen as an authority figure—including the clinician.

Although the main focus of therapy is the client himself, the parents' role within the partnership is still of critical importance, particularly with the child who has not achieved sufficient independence to be fully responsible for making his own decisions.

Locus of control

'Locus of control' is generally defined as the degree to which a person perceives a causal relationship between his own behaviour and its consequences. Locus of control theory suggests that it is possible to gauge an individual's attitude to his environment on a continuum between two categories. This construct attempts to measure the extent to which a person perceives events as being a consequence of his or her own behaviour and therefore potentially under personal control (Lefcourt, 1976). If the relationship between outcome and response is perceived to be the result of personal effort or ability then the belief is labelled *internal control* and conversely, if the relationship is attributed to luck or to another person, then the belief is labelled *external control* (Rotter, 1966).

The development of internal control (i.e. responsibility for own actions, control of the environment) has been well researched and links have been found with the style of parenting adopted. Lefcourt (1982) discusses familial determinants and influences on a child's locus of control. The maintenance of a warm, supportive, positive relationship between parent and child, interspersed with parental encouragement seems more likely to foster a child's belief and the development of internal control than is a relationship characterised by punishment, rejection, and criticism.

A study by Chandler et al. (1980) demonstrated that parents of 'internals' were less authoritarian but more authoritative, and more accepting and rewarding of independence than parents of 'externals'.

Lefcourt (1982) summarises the issues by suggesting that:

> both pampered and neglected children, then, through lack of experience with contingent reinforcement, may fail to explore and discover the relationship between acts and outcomes from which beliefs in the order of causal sequences develop.

Studies in the area of locus of control strongly support clinical experience that extreme protectiveness by the parents minimises the expectation of the child that he can exert some control over his environment.

We feel that this issue is particularly relevant to the family with an adolescent who stutters. It would seem likely that the more 'external' the adolescent is, the less he will feel in control of his own destiny. He will see life events, stresses and anxieties as being a matter of chance. He is more likely to look to his parents or professionals to initiate changes, confounding his problem even further and most likely supplementing difficulties which are already present in his environment.

Locus of control as a dimension of social skills

There is evidence that locus of control is an important area in the development of adequate social skills functioning. Trower, Bryant and Argyle (1978) discussed situational determinants of behaviour by use of the locus of control approach. The problem of inadequate social–situational adaptation was considered in terms of the internal–external dimensions related to degree of control over events. The authors go on to speculate that a causal circle exists between failure to produce appropriate adaptive behaviour and a disbelief in the ability to influence life events.

We consider that social skills training addresses the issues of locus of control very effectively. The hypothesis is that the more responsibility the client takes for his own actions/therapy/progress, the more likely he is to achieve success. The more external the locus of control, the stronger the client's attitude will be of 'victim' with little control of life events and less choice.

An intensive fluency course for adults was conducted by Craig, Franklin and Andrews (1984). These researchers showed that those externally oriented subjects whose scores, on the locus of control scale, did not change towards internality were more likely to relapse. Further research suggested that the locus of control can be therapeutically altered and the results demonstrated that fluency was maintained and relapse prevented (Craig and Andrews, 1985).

Summary

The aim of this chapter has been to discuss the complexity of the issues concerning the adolescent who stutters. It is clearly important to have a theoretical framework for understanding the development of stuttering within the context of the transition from childhood to adulthood. Therefore, we have included an overview of pertinent theories and models concerning the development of stammering and related these to adolescence. The central issues of self-image, social skills, locus of control and parental involvement have been discussed and will be elaborated on as part of the asssessment and therapy process. Successful management depends upon an extensive assessment of the physical, environmental, developmental and psychological factors of stuttering and this is addressed in the following chapter.

Chapter 2
The Assessment of the Adolescent Who Stutters

> The period of adolescence is exciting and creative, yet it can be tumultuous and volatile. There are a considerable number of developmental hurdles that challenge the emotional and physical stability of adolescents themselves and also those who are in charge of their care, such as their family and the community system.
>
> (Oster et al., 1988)

If we accept the notion of adolescence as the transitional period from childhood to adulthood, which brings with it the demands and pressures of relatively rapid physiological development and concomitant emotional, psychological and cognitive changes, it is clear that assessment of an individual who is entering into this phase is a highly complex, challenging task.

The essence of adolescence, it can be argued, is change. Not only change within the individual, as cited above, but change in the perceptions of that individual by others; namely, parents, family and, indeed, society at large. Erikson (1968) sees adolescence as the phase of identity formation. How the individual's identity develops is a direct result of a complex interaction between two major psycho-social stressors—the development of 'self' and constraints imposed by 'society'. The interplay between the changes in internal demands (e.g. libido, the need for independence, aggression/dominance) and external pressures (expectations of parents, peers, societal rules, etc.) are defined and redefined by the individual, moulded and modified by experience over time. The individual's relative success or failure in reconciling these internal and external demands will ultimately influence his emergence into stable adulthood. Consequently, practitioners in the field generally accept that effective assessment of adolescents must go beyond merely focusing on the skills and deficits of the individual. A number of authors (Haley, 1973, 1980; Minuchin, 1974; Watzlawick, 1984; Rustin, 1991) assert that in order to gain real insight into the world of the adolescent it is imperative that the clinician has an in-depth understanding of the family history and dynamics, as well as the subject's social milieu.

It can be appreciated that this approach is particularly relevant to the adolescent who stutters. By virtue of the problem of stuttering itself, there will invariably be issues arising from the case history involving communication, relationships and self-image which are of concern to the young person who stutters and may influence his effective transition into adulthood.

Within this chapter we present a case history format which we have found useful in the diagnostic interviewing of adolescents who stutter and their families. We provide some practical guidance for the clinician which, through experience, we feel is of particular relevance when approaching this task with adolescents. The case history is not intended as a tool which will provide the clinician with 'all the answers'. From this initial interview there may follow other indicators which will point to the need for further, specific investigations. We shall also be proposing some examples of additional assessment tools which may be appropriate.

The case history may be viewed as the starting point, which allows the results of any further assessment to be placed within a functional context. Moreover, it is likely that, having gained an initial impression of the adolescent's world, the speech and language clinician will enhance this knowledge and understanding throughout the therapeutic management of the client and his family; re-evaluating and adjusting the focus on the initial information gained.

The interview procedure

Following referral to our Centre for Stammering Children, we stipulate that *both* parents (with the exception of single-parent families) attend the consultation interview (Rustin and Cook, 1995). This sets the foundation for the long-term working relationship between the parents, the client and the clinician.

It is appropriate in some circumstances to offer a preliminary interview to the family to ascertain their willingness, availability and commitment to enter the full assessment. At this stage it is explained that the procedure requires $3-3\frac{1}{2}$ hours from both the client and the parents; that the purpose is to offer a comprehensive interview in order to gain a detailed picture of the adolescent within the context of the family and that management recommendations can only be made following the full consultation. Clinicians may often feel pressurized into commencing therapy before they have an adequate understanding of all the issues concerning a particular family. In our opinion it is better not to embark on therapy that is unlikely to succeed, as many years of unsuccessful therapy have a debilitating effect on clients who stutter and clinicians alike. We have found that when parents understand the importance of their role, they willingly commit themselves to work as part of a team approach for the long-term benefit of their child.

Where practicable, we would suggest a team of two speech and language therapists working concurrently. One will be responsible for the adolescent interview and assessment, whereas the other completes the parental interview. The formulation of the management plan is based on the findings from both clinicians, although the clinician who interviews the parents will take overall responsibility for the management plan. Where staffing is not available for this dual clinic, we recommend that the adolescent's interview is completed before the parental consultation, but that both appointments are arranged simultaneously and within a few days of each other. It is important that summing up and feedback are completed with parents and the adolescent together.

The first stage—setting the scene

It should be remembered that many adolescents who stutter may not be attending an assessment entirely of their own volition. Often, it is the concerns of the parents or carers which has precipitated the initial referral for specialist advice. Although this may not always be the case, the speech and language therapist should be aware of this possibility and undertake certain strategies to defuse any potential antagonism or anxiety on the part of the adolescent client. There are a number of significant principles in approaching the interview procedure which are of particular relevance to the parents of adolescent clients. Rustin and Cook (1983) stress the importance of establishing a rapport with the family before the clinician attempts to elicit information from them. In practical terms, this means observing social gestures, such as greetings and introductions, offering refreshments, enquiring about journeys to the clinic and information about the department and clinicians conducting the interview. An outline of the structure of the ensuing session is provided and an explanation given to all parties that, although the parents and teenager will be interviewed separately in the first instance, there will be the opportunity to meet together at the end of the session in order to make decisions regarding the way forward. This will serve to minimise anxiety on the part of the parents and the young adult in relationship to secrecy or hidden agendas and also establishes the role of the clinician.

Weins and Matarazzo (1983) endorse this view and stress the importance of a prompt start to the interview in order to avoid the build up of anxiety or antagonism on the part of the client and parents. The clinician should provide clear, accurate introductions to him- or herself and to any colleagues involved in the interview. Simple issues, such as how the client should address you and how he wishes to be addressed should be clarified. The adolescent should be addressed directly, not via parents or carers, although it is important that they also feel included in the initial dialogue. Overall, the clinician should stress that the adolescent will be fully involved in any decision-making process following interview, in order to that he or she may be established as a prime mover in any future management and to acknowledge that, ultimately, it is the adolescent's problem and that he may influence the final choices regarding future management strategies. Having ensured that all have understood the procedure, the interview should begin.

The diagnostic interview

It is vital that the adolescent has trust in the interviewer and in the diagnostic interviewing process. As Oster et al. (1988) suggest, many adolescents may be wary of unfamiliar adults and it is therefore important to offer straightforward communication about problem areas. In our experience, however, once trust has been gained, many teenagers find the opportunity to talk directly about fears, worries or concerns to an unbiased, non-judgmental adult highly rewarding. The importance, therefore, of establishing the initial rapport with the adolescent who stutters cannot be overemphasised. For example, in order to encourage self-disclosure and hence gain clearer insights, it is essential that an ambience of mutual respect, trust and confidentiality is achieved, which will largely arise out of the adolescent's initial impression of the interviewer. One 16-year-old client attending our clinic, who initially presented as an anxious, rather taciturn interviewee, became increasingly forthcoming as the interview proceeded. When asked, towards the end of the interview, whether he felt we might be of help to him he replied, *'Yes, because this is the first time I've done all the talking, usually, the therapists just tell me what they think is best'*.

The fluency assessment

This phase of the initial interview is a relatively non-emotive, straightforward procedure and the client may be familiar with aspects of its content if he has received speech and language therapy in the past. The clinician should provide a brief outline and explanation of the structure of the assessment to reassure the youngster that he is not being 'tested', as this can adversely affect performance. The fluency interview should be audiotaped and videotaped wherever possible. We have found that the quality of audiotape recording is enhanced by a clip-on lapel microphone.

Our fluency assessment comprises seven speaking situations: automatic speech; echoic speech; reading; naming; monologue; asking and answering questions, and engaging in conversation. The format for the assessment has been clearly outlined in *The Assessment and Therapy Programme for Dysfluent Children* (Rustin, 1987a) and is reproduced in Appendix I.

The fluency assessment will yield a measure of number of stuttered words per minute (SW/M), percentage of stuttered words (%SW) and words spoken per minute (WS/M) during the observed period. Types of stuttering behaviour are also noted, including whole-word and part-word repetitions, prolongations, struggle and other behaviours, such as avoidance, concomitant physical gestures and so on. Results from this assessment constitute a baseline which contributes to planning and evaluating therapy. Further measures of the stuttering behaviour should be made periodically in order to evaluate changes in the degree and type of stuttering. This represents one aspect of progress. Following the fluency assessment, when the client is often more relaxed and comfortable with the therapist, the case history will be taken. We always reiterate that we will be sharing the results of the assessment with the young adult at the end of the session.

The case history

The case history (Appendix II) is structured to allow for the gradual investigation of the client's personal world—his stresses and pressures, his skills and pleasures. The first section is aimed at gaining insight into the speech problem and is largely factual, seeking the adolescent's viewpoint.

Section A: Speech

Present complaint

Here the adolescent is given the opportunity to state the problem as he sees it. It may be that the individual does not view the dysfluency as the central problem in his world which will give the clinician valuable insight into the relative importance of the stutter and the client's potential motivation within therapy.

The clinician needs to establish whether the teenager has any perception of his own stuttering behaviour and its ontogenesis. Conture (1982) states that the clearer the individual's understanding of his problem, the more likely he is to find a solution. Therefore, it is worth investigating how the stutterer feels that the dysfluency is manifested and whether he is aware of any patterns affecting the behaviour. Furthermore, questioning should establish whether the client has his own theories about the cause and nature of the problem. This can yield helpful information about the client's perception of his own ability to affect the behaviour and to exert control over it, which may have implications for future management. Questions relating to the client's own strategies for dealing with the dysfluency extend this insight further, as do later questions regarding the client's own feelings about the differing reactions of others to his stutter. As the interview progresses, the questioning becomes gradually more personal, less factual. This is in order to encourage the teenager to become accustomed to the process of disclosure; initially of unemotive information, eventually moving into more sensitive areas. After an episode of personal disclosure, the interview reverts to less emotive issues, such as general health and hospital admissions. This is intended to allow the interviewee and interviewer to proceed at a comfortable pace and to prevent the client feeling overexposed.

Section B: School

There follows a section which is broadly related to issues concerning the client's experiences of school life. Any comprehensive case history for adolescents must take account of their academic and social functioning within school (Blotcky, 1984).

Gaining the teenager's opinions and impressions of his school, teachers and peers may reveal a great deal about his relative social adjustment, his ability to cope with authority and authority figures (teachers), his problem-solving strategies and ability to adjust to social demands, and to integrate successfully. The individual's relationships with teachers need to be explored. In our experience this is an issue which can be a source of great strength for a teenager or, conversely, one of considerable anxiety. Invariably, it is an issue about which the adolescent has a great deal to say when confidentiality is assured. We have had many reports from clients who have found the help and support received from an understanding teacher invaluable in their educational progress and personal growth. Equally, however, we have also received reports of unenlightened teachers who appear to have little or no understanding of the painful experiences of the person with a stutter. Indeed, their actions can serve to exacerbate the problem.

One 14-year-old client, who frequently played truant from his English classes, reported that his teacher would make him stand in front of the rest of his class to read a passage from an exam text. The boy would invariably stutter severely, whereupon it was usual practice for the teacher to mimic his stutter to the rest of the class before telling him to sit down with obvious disgust. However, the same 14-year-old excelled at French, where his teacher had discussed his speech problem openly with the boy and had agreed a management strategy with him which allowed him to volunteer to read out in class when he felt confident and able.

All such issues are highly pertinent and will have a bearing upon future management strategies in relationship to the dysfluency. At a simple level, it may be necessary for the speech and language clinician to arrange for further assessment of specific skills, such as literacy or perceptual skills, if so indicated. We have explored the potential issues in this area in the final chapter of this book. However, of equal importance is the way the school deals with the dysfluent young person. There will often be an educational role for the clinician when revelations are gained about unhelpful management within this setting. The clinician should also investigate how the young person perceives his own performance at school. This may enlighten the interviewer about the teenager's own self-expectations and how far they approximate true ability.

Exams/qualifications

Questions relating to exams are of particular relevance, not least because this is a period in which ability is tested at regular intervals within the educational system. Some individuals may report heightened stress at such times, which may have an adverse affect upon their fluency.

School truancy and any deterioration in academic achievement, classroom conduct, incidence of bullying, either as victim or perpetrator are other areas which are explored directly within this section of the assessment. As Oster et al. (1988) point out, however, it may be necessary at a later stage to seek independent testimony of these issues as information from the individual or family may not be comprehensive. Permission to contact the school and gain such information should, of course, always be sought.

Sex education

The interview proceeds to investigate the adolescent's knowledge about and attitudes towards sex, as well as his experience. This is an area which, if handled sensitively but directly, the teenager will usually be quite happy to discuss. Whilst the clinician should maintain a non-pejorative attitude towards the information received, an awareness should be maintained of the adolescent's developmental stage, both physically and emotionally. As Oster et al. (1988) state 'continued sexual interactions for a 13-year-old may indicate maladaptive functioning, whilst this may not be so unusual for an adolescent of 18'.

It is also important for the clinician to be convinced of the necessity for asking about such personal issues and their relevance to future management of the dysfluent young person and to lay aside any personal embarrassment which may hinder the process of disclosure. The individual's developing attitudes and experiences of their own sexuality are highly prominent during the adolescent phase. Many teenagers have worries and fears about their own self-image which are of great concern. As one 16-year-old client put it, *'I'd really like to talk to girls, to have a regular girlfriend, but I know that if I started talking to one I'd just stutter and they'd think I was some weirdo, but anyway, because I don't talk to them, they all think I'm weird anyway—it's so frustrating.'* In our view, this is a convincing enough argument.

Peer relationships

The interview moves on to questions relating to friendships. This will yield information about the individual's relative integration or isolation in the social context. It is important to explore not only the range but the duration of friendships, the opportunities for social contact and regularity of that contact. Some teenagers may be keen to present themselves as popular, well-integrated individuals, but it is only with specific questioning that this representation is validated.

Social life

The section on social life serves to explore further the range of social activities to which the individual has access. There are also direct questions related to eating problems. It is generally held that eating disorders, such as anorexia nervosa or bulimia, start during adolescence and, in particular, although not exclusively, affect young girls. Harkaway (1987) says that eating disorders, including obesity, which commence during adolescence are often a result of a combination of complex interrelated psychological, behavioural, biological, ethnic and sociological sources of tension.

It can be argued that these tensions may also be present in the adolescent who stutters to greater or lesser degree. Indeed, our experience of interviewing many adolescents has led us to believe that eating disorders are more common than clinicians may suspect, particularly in female clients who often have a poor self-image. Hence, eating and nutrition is an important area which should not be overlooked in the diagnostic interview.

Questions relating to pocket money, allowances and wages establish the adolescent's relative financial independence from his parents. His ability to budget and control expenditure also gives insight into his maturity and social competence.

Section C: Home

This section of the interview is broadly related to the home environment, family relationships, discipline and personal habits. Here, the assessment reverts to an episode of relatively unemotive questioning, for reasons previously outlined.

Sleeping arrangements and personal responsibilities within the home can, however, be illuminating. One client, the eldest child in an overcrowded household, was required to sleep on the family couch. This was an issue of which school and social services were apparently unaware, but one which helped to explain why this young man would habitually fall asleep during afternoon lessons at school. This is an important area as, apart from the psychological effects of such extreme situations, fatigue is often a key element in deteriorating fluency in adolescents.

Later in this section, we ask directly about bedtime routines with essentially the same purpose in mind. Conflict with parents or carers regarding regulations for bedtime may often be an issue causing a great deal of unresolved tension within the family. Zarb (1992) cites disrupted sleeping patterns as a typical symptom of a depressed adolescent.

The teenager's role, if any, in sharing household tasks, also demonstrates the degree of responsibility expected and accepted by him and can provide valuable insight, which may be relevant to proposed management strategies.

Siblings

An exploration of the client's relationship with his siblings may give information into sources of support, tension or conflict within the family.

Parents

The interview begins to delve into the adolescent's relationship with his parents and his perception of their relationship with each other, where appropriate. Some teenagers may find this a difficult area to discuss initially as they are worried that what they have to say may be disclosed to their parents. Often, the adolescent may be protective of his parents, not wishing to seem to betray their trust. Hence, it is important that the clinician reassures the client that what he has to say will not be divulged to his parents and is in confidence.

Blotcky (1984) feels that direct questioning about family relationships and events as well as how the adolescent views himself within the family, are vital elements of the diagnostic interview and should not be avoided. Handled sensitively, this will lead to a clearer understanding of the youngster's situation.

Discipline

Questions about discipline within the family home are highly pertinent. It is important to discover whether methods of punishment and discipline are age-appropriate, consistently applied and effective from the point of view of the adolescent.

Fenwick and Smith (1993) assert 'sanctions should never be demeaning, and physical punishment should never be used against a young adult'. This may be the ideal but, in our experience, it is not always what happens and will influence any recommendations the speech and language therapist makes regarding management of the dysfluency problem.

Restrictions on friends, reading materials, television or video viewing can be the source of much antagonism between teenagers and their parents and should be explored.

It is necessary to establish the adolescent's experiences, either past or present, with regard to drugs/substance abuse, alcohol and cigarettes. This again can be a difficult area for disclosure and it is important that the clinician should maintain a non-judgmental manner when following this line of questioning. It is essential information, however, as it will inform about any behavioural/conduct problems which may be being demonstrated by the individual, as well as highlighting unhealthy peer group pressures from which the teenager is finding it difficult to extricate himself.

If the clinician is soliciting such information, however, she must also be prepared to deal with issues which arise from the disclosure: for example, helping the young person to tell his family about the problem and guiding him to appropriate support agencies if appropriate. We have noted the increasing numbers of young people who have had either direct or indirect experience of drugs and/or alcohol. Wright and Pearl's (1986) longitudinal study showed a sharp increase in the proportion of teenagers who had been offered drugs and whose contemporaries were taking illicit drugs. It is an area which requires investigation and one which should never be overlooked in a comprehensive behavioural assessment targeted at this age group.

Section D: Concepts

The penultimate section of direct questions in the interview looks at the individual's concepts of self. Questions relating to best and worst life experiences can take some time to evoke answers, as it may be something to which the individual has given little thought. This line of questioning may be demanding in that it requires a decision about a range of possible life experiences which the young adult may find confusing or which may still be unresolved. Similarly, it can be difficult for some teenagers, without a clear sense of self, to think of three good things about their personalities, but they may identify three 'bad' things quite readily.

Investigation of fears and phobias, response to personal failure, degree of empathy for the predicaments of others as well as problem-solving strategies, adds to our knowledge of the individual's coping strategies.

The last question in this section seeks to discover the one thing the individual would most like to change about his life. This can be a very enlightening exercise, not only for the clinician but also the interviewee. Although one might expect the response *'My stutter'* this is by no means the only response and can be of great assistance to both parties in placing a perspective upon the relative importance of the dysfluency problem in the life of the individual.

Section E: Speech and language therapy

The final section of the interview moves back, initially, into more factual territory regarding the individual's previous experience of speech and language therapy and his perception of its relative effectiveness. This will give a very useful insight into the teenager's expectations of the clinician and the therapeutic process. A key question in this section relates to the client's perception of his life without a stutter. This gives important insights into the client's investment in the stutter. We have found that many young people believe that if only their stutter would disappear their lives would be perfect in all respects. For example, a 16-year-old who had been in trouble with the police and was the subject of threats from peers, with a forthcoming court appearance pending, reported that if only he could get rid of his stutter his life would get back on to an even path! Clearly, in such instances, unrealistic expectations such as these would need to be addressed to enable the adolescent to place the dysfluency into a more reasonable perspective.

Finally, an opportunity is given to the adolescent to disclose any further information to the interviewer or to ask any questions.

Section F: Client's reaction to interview

This is a descriptive section of the assessment which gives the clinician the opportunity to make comments on the overall presentation of the client during interview. This includes observation of concomitant behaviours, evidence of avoidance and his social communication skills as demonstrated throughout the interview and assessment process.

Section G: Modification of stuttering behaviour

This section allows the clinician and client to explore aspects of speech modification which the client may find helpful in the achievement of improved fluency. (Note: a detailed description of the fluency-enhancing strategies: Easy Onset; Flow of Speech; Breath Control; Soft Contacts, and Relaxation, which we employ with adolescents is presented in Chapter 4 of this book.)

Language assessments

The *British Picture Vocabulary Scale* (Dunn et al., 1982) is routinely administered as an formal assessment of the individual's current abilities in the comprehension of vocabulary. The *Test of Adolescent Word Finding* (German, 1990) also offers significant information in determining other possible contributory factors underpinning the nature of the dysfluency.

In conclusion, it is usual for us to present a brief explanation including some facts and figures about stuttering, incidence rates, sex ratios, historical perspectives, research into causation and so on. This is presented simply and factually and we have found that it is an aspect of the interview which young adults often find helpful and reassuring, as it may be the first time that they have been given this information directly (Appendix III).

The parental interview

We have previously given our view that adolescents need to be viewed as individuals who function in a range of contexts, e.g. family, schools, with the opposite sex, with peers, within the establishment. Therefore, in order to understand the adolescent fully we need to understand how he functions within those contexts. This is a generally accepted approach within the fields of social psychology and behavioural science (Coleman and Hendry, 1990; Erikson, 1968; Oster et al., 1988; Rustin, 1987). However, the area of in-depth investigation of family issues can be challenging for the speech and language clinician, who may feel insecure or unconvinced of the need to delve into such sensitive areas of their client's world. Our own view is that a clinician will be unable to facilitate positive, sustainable change for an adolescent client unless the dynamics of the family have been investigated and understood. All of the related literature on the nature of adolescence indicates the complexity of the changing relationships between parents and the emerging young adult. Given the issues touched upon earlier regarding the importance of developing self-image, of relationships and demands and capacities during the adolescent phase of life, we feel that it is vital that the speech and language clinician working with such clients is fully equipped to make this area of practice as effective as possible.

Rustin (1987) has produced a detailed parental interview which has been used for several years with parents of children who stutter. This interview procedure has been outlined in detail in that programme and we will not attempt to review the whole procedure again here. We have found that the assessment provides a useful framework for interviewing parents of adolescents who stutter, with little adaptation necessary (Appendix IV).

At the beginning of the parental interview, the clinician should continue the process of reassurance which began with the family's arrival at the clinic. Parents may feel that the purpose of the exercise is to find fault with them or their child's upbringing and it is important to allay these fears from the outset. We always point out to parents that there are no right or wrong answers to the questions that we are about to ask and that we recognise that each may offer a different point of view. We explain that this is why we stipulate that both parents, where present within the family unit, must attend the family interview, in order that we can gain a holistic view of the family and their management of the problem. Furthermore, we reassure them that there is no evidence that parents cause stammering in their children and, indeed, it is likely that much of what they do is helpful. We explain that they are under no obligation to answer all questions if they do not wish to do so and that they will be given ample opportunity to ask questions at the end of the session. Oster et al. (1988) suggest that it is important during the subsequent phase of the interview, to strike a balance between asking questions that will provide information and allowing the parents some opportunity to 'tell their story'. This will help to ascertain the level of uniformity of views between both parents and their own views about any problems within the family and how they deal with them. McGoldrick and Gerson (1985), Rustin (1987) and Peters and Guitar (1991) all stress the importance of identifying the presenting complaint and the need to gain each parent's view of the problem.

The purpose of the parental interview, in combination with the adolescent's interview, is largely to define the function of the dysfluency within the family context and the role of the adolescent in relation to his family. The closing phase of the interview must also be handled in a sensitive and organised manner. It is of paramount importance that the clinician should actively lead this phase above all others. Once the line of questioning within the parental interview is completed, we provide a short but direct outline of information about dysfluency, similar to that offered to the young adults in their interview.

The clinician should then take a break in order to gather information from the adolescent interview, including the fluency assessment and other assessments, as appropriate. Once this is completed, the clinician presents a summary to the parents of the information gathered from their own and their child's interview. This is an opportunity to emphasise to the parents their crucial role in helping the young adult to develop his strategies for dealing with his problem. We reiterate that stuttering is not caused by parents. It may be the case that the parents have exacerbated the problem through unhelpful strategies of their own, but as Peters and Guitar (1991) stress, there is little point in making an issue of this if you wish them to change their practice into something which is ultimately more productive.

At this point, the clinician may outline to the parents the recommendations regarding future management that seem appropriate at this stage. However, it is vital that the young adult is included in this discussion as soon as possible and no decisions should be made without his direct involvement and agreement. As Peters and Guitar (1991) point out, the regrouping of the family following separate interviews is an important time as it serves to show the young adult that we consider him able to work independently from his parents and it also demonstrates to the parents that they can assume a supportive rather than directive role.

Above all, the final phase of the interview must be well organised, and recommendations must be clear, concise, rationalised and measurable. Agreement to recommendations should be gained from each family member and a method of recording progress provided, for example, through homework sheets. It should be the responsibility of all family members involved in the recommendations to undertake to complete tasks and to forward feedback to the clinician as appropriate. More detailed examples of how we approach this task are provided in Chapter 3 of this book. It is only through such direct, honest approaches, enhanced by active listening and focusing on the information presented to the clinician, that acceptance of any recommendations will be achieved. This first introduction to diagnostic interviewing will, if successful, set the scene for future intervention with the dysfluent teenager and will ensure that the whole family is actively supporting rather than unknowingly counteracting the therapeutic regime.

Further assessments

Whilst the above diagnostic interview procedures will complete the initial phase of assessment, it is usually the case that further in-depth assessment will be required as a part of the ongoing therapeutic process, once a young adult is accepted for treatment. This fact should be clearly explained to the teenager and his parent(s).

It is an accepted part of clinical practice for the clinician to re-evaluate therapy in order to confirm that the client is on the appropriate track and continuing to make progress. In order to measure such variables, it is important for the clinician to take account of those aspects of communicative competence which are important to the client himself, as well as his attitudes and feelings about his own level of competence measured against that of others in his world. We have outlined below a broad range of assessment tools we have found useful. Furthermore, we have developed our own assessment procedure relating to social skills which contributes to the management plan (Appendix V).

Research, cited in Chapter 1, indicates the relatively high coincidence of other speech and language difficulties in stuttering children and there may be a need to investigate such difficulties in the young adult. However, this area has been dealt with in the final chapter of this book and we will only attempt here to focus on those areas which we feel have immediate relevance to the teenager who is dysfluent.

Attitudes and self-perceptions

The *Modified Erikson Scale, S-24* (Andrews and Cutler, 1974) seeks to obtain information about the client's perceptions of and attitudes towards his dysfluency by asking him to judge his communicative competence against a series of 24 separate statements. For example, 'Even the idea of giving a talk in public makes me afraid'. The client will make a subjective judgement as to whether this and the other statements are true or false in his own case.

The clinician is then able to gain a relative measure of the client's self-perception as a communicator which is very helpful in establishing the need for therapy targeted at improving this area. Guitar and Bass (1978) have suggested that changes in attitude during treatment are related to the effectiveness of therapy and long-term outcomes. Our own experience with a significant number of adolescents who stutter certainly supports this finding.

Another questionnaire which clinicians may find helpful with this client group is the *Stutterer's Self Rating Scale of Reactions to Speech Situations* (Johnson, Darley and Spriestersbach, 1952). These avoidance scales, which are quite exhaustive, attempt to assess the client's tendency to avoid situations, a total of 40 being provided. This assessment is particularly useful with adolescent clients as so many of the situations are pertinent to this age group. However, we have found that the rating scale can be difficult to explain to younger teenagers.

Woolf's (1967) *Perceptions of Stuttering Inventory* (PSI) can also be useful with some clients. It is a lengthy questionnaire which focuses the client into the characteristics of his stuttering behaviour, as well as his communication style and some reference to avoidance of specific speaking situations. It can be a useful tool, particularly with those clients who appear to have little awareness of their own stammering behaviour and its functions and effects.

Such questionnaires, although they may initially appear quite time-consuming, may, if used with appropriate clients, prove very effective as initial steps in a therapeutic regime which has a focus on attitude change. They can assist the therapist in structuring her own plans as well as providing replicable parameters in order to measure change periodically. (See p.32 on outcome measures.)

The *Personal Questionnaire Rapid Scaling Technique* (PQRST) (Mulhall, 1977): this assessment offers a standardised measure of the client's attitudes towards a variety of personal speaking situations where difficulties occur. Apart from offering a test/retest opportunity for monitoring change in attitude and behaviour, the information gained from this questionnaire is used in the second week of our intensive therapy course to identify individual speaking situations which need to be explored, reconstrued and practised.

Social communication skills

This important aspect of interpersonal functioning has been shown to influence the ability to maintain fluency following therapy (Rustin, 1984; Rustin and Kuhr, 1989). Other specialists in the field of social skills (Adams, Shea and Kacerguis, 1978; Anderson and Messick, 1974; Greenberger and Sorenson,1974) have postulated three underlying social dimensions which, taken together, constitute a comprehensive definition of the necessary social competencies which enable an individual to integrate successfully with peers. These are:

1. Social knowledge: the ability to adapt or recognise appropriate emotional states in relationship to specific social contexts.
2. Empathy: the ability to empathise with and understand the viewpoint of others.
3. Locus of control: a sense of self-initiation and control over one's own actions and destiny.

We will return later in this chapter to an examination of locus of control and its interplay with empathic abilities within teenagers as this has particular relevance in our view to the successful treatment of adolescents who stutter.

We approach the assessment of social skills by use of the hierarchy put forward by Rustin and Kuhr (1989). This hierarchy comprises seven discrete skills: observation; listening; turntaking; negotiation; relaxation; praise and reinforcement, and problem-solving. Assessment of an individual's competence against these parameters through observation and direct questioning constitutes an initial baseline from which the therapist and client can work together to improve the client's skill base. A checklist of social skills (Appendix V) is completed and shared with the client where appropriate. Direct questioning is carried out by means of a simple rating scale (Appendix VI) which asks the client to rate his relative skill in areas such as eye-contact, listening, initiation and maintenance of conversation, proximity, praise and reinforcement, assertiveness, problem-solving and rate of speech. We have found this to be an extremely useful way of cueing adolescents into these important parameters of communication and enabling them to become more objective about their own skills, particularly if used in conjunction with video recordings. Clearly, such measures are highly subjective in nature. We feel that this is entirely appropriate, however, as an individual's social competence is in itself a subjective paradigm which will vary across time and from one witness to another. In a later chapter, we will discuss how this framework can be applied within intensive group and individual therapy.

Locus of control

Since the initial and extensive research by Lefcourt (1966) and Rotter

(1966) into the field of locus of control, there has been a significant growth of interest in the application of this theoretical framework to assessment and measurement of therapeutic outcomes. Locus of control has been defined as the degree to which an individual can perceive a causal relationship between his own behaviour or actions and ultimate consequences or reward. The theory presupposes that this aspect of social functioning will vary both between and within individuals, across situations and over time. Adams (1983) studied the social competency (including locus of control) of male and female adolescents aged 14, 15, 17 and 18 years and found significant age and sex differences in levels of locus of control within the sample. Many questionnaires have now been developed in an attempt to measure an individual's perception of his ability to exert control over his world. Rotter (1966); Lifschitz (1973); Lefcourt (1976); Nowicki and Strickland (1973) and Craig and Andrews (1985) approach this task in essentially the same way—by individuals placing themselves on a locus of control construct scale or continuum, which has two poles: 'internally controlled' and 'externally controlled'. An individual who is placed at the internal end of the spectrum is somebody who feels in control of his environment, able to affect outcomes or events through his own actions or efforts. The externally controlled individual is somebody who feels at the mercy of fate, luck or the actions of powerful others in his environment, unable to exert personal influence over his own destiny.

Although the major proportion of research into locus of control has been carried out with adults and children rather than adolescents there are striking themes recurring within this theoretical framework which have direct relevance to the assessment and treatment of this age group. For example, the degree to which the young adult feels that he is able to exert some influence over his dysfluency, and the extent to which this, in turn, precludes him from participating in a variety of social situations, are issues which will be recognised by the speech and language clinician working with this client group. One 17-year-old client in our clinic, during the assessment phase of his treatment programme, volunteered that he felt that the stutter was in control of him rather than him having any control of it. Consequently, he felt that he had become socially isolated, felt awkward with people of his own age and avoided conversations because he 'couldn't take the chance of it suddenly catching me out'. This experience is supported by the research of Adam (1983) which demonstrated a positive relationship between peer group popularity and social competence. The young man in question, although highly intelligent and with a quantatively moderate stutter, had failed to develop age-appropriate social skills, felt isolated and frustrated and could not see any way of influencing this situation himself. Upon assessment of his locus of control he was strongly 'external'.

Within our clinic we use a locus of control questionnaire (Craig,

Franklin and Andrews, 1984). It consists of 17 statements, six of which strongly indicate 'internal control', the remaining 11 being 'external' in nature. The respondent is asked to choose his own level of agreement with each statement from a 6-point scale, ranging from 'strongly disagree' through to 'strongly agree'. Once completed, a transposition of scores for the internal questionnaire items is carried out. These, taken together with scores for the external items, yield a measure of relative internality/externality; the higher the score gained the more externally controlled the individual.

This assessment has important implications, in our view, for planning appropriate therapeutic regimes and for gauging outcomes of therapy. Spence and Spence (1980) have emphasised the importance of facilitating the development of social skills by including a focus on the necessary cognitive/attitude changes required in the individual, such as improved self-esteem and locus of control. We feel, therefore, that an investigation of locus of control, taken with assessment of social skills, is of equal importance to an accurate measure of levels of dysfluency within the initial phase of intervention.

Speech and language clinicians working with teenagers who stutter will be aware of the sensitivity and complexity of their work. In this chapter we have emphasised the importance of effective and appropriate assessment strategies which will ultimately yield adequately detailed information to allow for incisive and productive treatment planning. However, assessment is clearly an ongoing process. The rate and degree of change within the young adult population is so striking and so rapid that it requires the therapist to constantly revisit hypotheses about an individual case.

Outcome measures

The measurement of progress and outcome is seen as important for a number of reasons:

* Clients, as partners in the process of change, need to have identifiable targets and goals to acquire the self-monitoring skills which are the foundations of long-term success.
* Ongoing measurements allow the therapist and client to modify therapy as necessary. For example, a comparison of findings in the clinical setting with the client's self-rating of outside situations will ascertain whether transfer of skills is taking place.
* Measurement has the therapeutic effect of providing the client with consistent and accurate information about his progress. For example, a client who reports that he is making no headway will be able to see from his homework diary the changes that have already been achieved. The accumulation of this information provides valuable insight to the client.

• Regular measurements ensure that therapist and client remain focused on agreed treatment goals.

In addition to the client-centred needs for monitoring progress accurately, healthcare professionals within the British NHS are increasingly being required to audit, at every level, the quality of service provision for patients. Measures of outcome provide the essential information on treatment efficacy which justify therapeutic approaches.

This chapter has identified the assessments that we use at initial interview, as well as other measures and reassessments which may be taken periodically throughout and at the end of therapy. We have divided these measurements into three categories which can be plotted on the communication skills chart in Appendix VII. This offers a simple visual display to illustrate overall targets in therapy, the individual's baseline measures and a personal profile of achievements. Each subsection is divided into a 5-point scale. A score of 1, at the centre of the circle, representing the 'severe' end of the scale with a score of 5 as the target outcome. In some categories there are more formal measures, whereas in others it is intentionally subjective. Training of therapists, within teams, in the use of these assessments is, however, extremely important in order to optimise inter-rater reliability. We are currently piloting this format and, as with all aspects of therapy, this will be revised and updated with experience.

Appendix VIII describes in detail the way scores are assigned within each category.

Category One: Verbal

Stutter

The quantity of stuttering is gained from the tape-recorded speech samples. We have elected to place >20% stuttering at the 'most severe' end of the scale, with >3% as the 'least severe'. (We do not consider that this measure is ever useful by itself.)

Types

A score of 1 is assigned when the most disruptive types of stuttering are present, for example, repetitions + prolongations + struggle + concomitants. However, a score of 5 would imply that the speech contained 'normal non-fluencies', for example, word repetitions, occasional syllable repetitions, pauses, reiterations, incomplete phrases, etc. with no signs of tension.

Avoidances

The client's verbal report is essential for assigning scores in this section.

A score of 1 would indicate that word avoidance is used persistently and in most situations, whereas a score of 5 would describe a client who always attempts the word he wishes, even if stuttering is the result. This particular aspect is of value with clients who are 'covert' with their stuttering behaviours.

Speech rate

This aspect is measured from the audiotape-recorded speech samples. At present we have elected to count all words spoken, including stuttered words. This information, with the 'percentage' stuttered words and 'types' of stuttering behaviours offers a useful and broad description for baseline measures and subsequent changes within therapy.

Volume and intonation

These are subjective assessments, but nonetheless important aspects for ongoing measures during therapy. More objectivity can be gained through use of video-recording and second rater scores.

Self-rating

Here, the client is given the opportunity for scoring himself on the 5-point scale and is a useful discussion point in relation to the other sections.

Category Two: Non-verbal

Eye-contact

A score of 1 is assigned to a client who generally has poor eye-contact, whether in the speaker or listener role. The scores are then graded towards more appropriate use of eye-contact, with 5 being 'normal' within all situations.

Observation

Again, a subjective measure whereby 1 would indicate a client's observation skills to be self-centred with little or no skill in observing other people. A score of 5 would be assigned when the client is able to make useful, competent and objective observations of situations. This frequently links with eye-contact.

Listening

Scores are assigned according to therapists' observations of the client's apparent listening skills. A score of 1 would denote a person who is distracted, appearing not to listen or clearly not listening, whereas 5 would be given to a client who shows clear evidence of listening which is adaptive to the social context.

Turntaking

A score of 1 would be given to a client who either interrupts inappropriately, does not allow interruptions or remains passive. Although this is another section which may appear very subjective, consensus between client and therapist will give a very useful indication and, again, videorecording is invaluable.

Mannerisms/tics

Although not appropriate in all clients, this can be an additional area for assessment. It would need to be defined in terms of speech or nonspeech related.

Facial expression

Again, consensus between therapists is important to assign scores at this level. The scoring is purposefully broad because of the possible range of deficit.

Self-rating

Here, the client is given the opportunity to evaluate his own skills.

Category Three: Cognitive–emotional

Locus of control

Although the locus of control questionnaire is a valuable tool for the therapist, the scores obtained are not directly transferable to these scales. They will offer guidelines which, when considered in the light of the client interview and self-evaluations, will enable a score to be assigned.

Situational avoidance

Again, the *Modified Erikson Scale, S-24,* will guide the scoring on this parameter, but we consider that it is valuable to obtain addition information from the client's viewpoint. A score of 1 will be characteristic of an individual who usually avoids stressful speaking situations, whereas 5 would indicate that a client will attempt all situations.

Self-esteem

Again, guidance can be gained from the PQRST and the Character Sketch (see pages 29 and 75), and the scores will be assigned as a result of the information gathered.

Problem-solving

Information for assigning scores in this section is obtained from the preceding information as well as the client's verbal report of his ability to solve problems in his daily life. For example, the strategies that he has developed for dealing with the stuttering, his description of how he deals with problems, who he relies on, his sources of information, his dependencies, or, indeed, his self-reliance.

Negotiation

Information for this section will commonly be obtained during the first few sessions of group therapy or in the individual family sessions. This is a particularly useful ongoing measure.

Assertiveness

Baseline scores will be assigned on the basis of the initial verbal report and re-assessed during the therapy programme.

Empathy

This section is similar to assertiveness, negotiation and problem-solving above. The baseline scores can be assigned from the interview, but will be constantly re-evaluated as part of the therapy process.

Self-rating

Another important opportunity for self-evaluation of the client's general understanding of the psychological aspects of the stuttering problem. This would be evaluated in terms of his understanding of the problem, his ability to construe the emotional aspects and whether he is able to take responsibility for the stuttering.

   In the subsequent chapter, we present our approach to structuring the information which has been gathered from assessments. This formulation is the essential starting point for developing appropriate treatment strategies.

Chapter 3
Planning Interventions

The speech and language clinician is above all a *practitioner*. Whilst the importance and value of objective assessment of communicative function and dysfunction has been widely accepted for many years within the profession, it is also generally recognised that to assess alone is not enough. This, by implication, means that the clinician is not only required to identify a problem but also to attempt to develop strategies in order to resolve that problem.

However, the task of placing the wide variety of potential assessment findings into a meaningful framework which will inform an hypothesis for intervention is rarely simple or straightforward. This fact is no less true for the clinician working with adolescents who stutter and their families. Such a professional may be faced with a complex web of inter-dependent factors, of greater or lesser degree, which are contributing to the maintenance of a (usually) chronic problem. Defining these factors will be a difficult process; selecting appropriate strategies to address such contributory elements adds to the task; yet perhaps the greatest challenge of all is to gain the compliance of the adolescent and his family in entering into the therapeutic process as active and cooperative participants.

We present in this chapter our approach to the evaluation and summarising of assessment information, the selection and development of intervention strategies and their underlying rationale. We have provided four case studies which we feel exemplify the application of this approach to a range of our teenage clients. In subsequent chapters, we elucidate upon the theoretical and philosophical basis to our 'communication skills approach' to intervention and explain how this can be applied within group intensive and individual service delivery options.

Rustin (1987) and Oster et al. (1988) both stress the importance of the clinician's leading role in closing the diagnostic interview with adolescents and their families. The clinician will be required to summarise information gathered in a concise and understandable manner, drawing together findings from the parental interview, adolescent interview and other diagnostic tools, such as the fluency assessment. The clinician's ability to present a structured, rational and acceptable treatment plan is of pivotal importance if the adolescent and his family are to be successfully engaged into the therapeutic process. Through our own experience, we have found that it is very helpful to have a structure which allows for the grouping of contributory elements under the following headings: Physiological factors; Cognitive–emotional factors; Behavioural factors, and Environmental factors. This allows the clinician to identify such elements and their relative importance in the overall picture of the presenting adolescent's problem and will, in turn, inform the decision-making process with regard to therapeutic intervention. We present below a grid (Figure 3.1) which we have found helpful in structuring our summary of issues arising from diagnostic interview. We suggest that clinicians may find this useful when feeding back to families following interview and when formulating intervention plans.

PHYSIOLOGICAL	COGNITIVE/EMOTIONAL
Family History Developmental History General Health Severity of Stutter (%, types, concomitants, avoidances, variability) Rates of speech Other learning difficulties Other:	Feeling about stuttering self image self expectations Internal/External locus of control Problem solving skills Empathy Attitude to parents Attitude to siblings Attitude to peers
BEHAVIOURAL	ENVIRONMENTAL
Antecedents of stuttering Consequences of stuttering Range of peer relationships Social communication skills Social functioning Academic performance Anti social behaviour Addictive behaviours Suicide attempts Eating Disorders Psychological Disorders	Family circumstances Physical Environment Parental Expectations Adolescent-Parental conflict Parent-parent conflict Position in family Sibling rivalry Turntaking in family parental rates of speech Cultural issues Bilingualism Peer Attitudes/Pressures School/College Expectations Other:

Figure 3.1 Grid summarising issues arising from diagnostic interview

Physiological factors

This section attempts to identify those issues which are essentially physiological in nature and which may be contributing to the maintenance of the problem. This includes family history of stuttering or other associated problems; the developmental history of the stuttering behaviour and other development; issues related to general health which may be felt to be exacerbating the speech problem; the adolescent's own rate of speech and the presence of any other learning difficulties, including dyslexia, higher level language problems, etc. Any other physiological issues which may arise should also be identified here.

Cognitive–emotional factors

Here we have attempted to isolate those issues which are personal to the adolescent himself; that is, his own feelings and attitudes about himself and others which may be contributing to the problem. This includes the teenager's feelings and attitudes towards his stuttering behaviour; self-image; self-expectations; locus of control, i.e. how able he feels to influence events in his life and to exert control over them; empathic abilities, i.e. his ability to appreciate and understand the feelings and viewpoints of others; his attitude towards his parents, siblings and peers and his relationships with them; his problem-solving skills; fear of failure and his relative assertiveness. The teenager's level of independence, both emotionally and financially, is also considered here.

Behavioural factors

In this section of the grid we have focused on those aspects of stuttering which are largely behavioural in nature. That is, how the dysfluency is manifested; precipitating (antecedents) and ensuing (consequences) factors; social competence, including specific speaking and social situations which are problematic for the young adult; the relative richness or paucity of peer group networks; academic performance; evidence of addictive behaviours; suicide attempts; eating disorders or any other psychological or adjustment problems.

Environmental factors

Here we take account of a wide range of external factors which may be influencing the adolescent and his presenting problem. Family circumstances, including financial problems, illness of family members, bereavement; physical environment, including whether the young adult has his own room, location of home, satisfaction with home circumstances; parental expectations of teenager; extended family expectations; evidence of parent–adolescent conflict or difficulties with discipline and management; evidence of parent–parent conflict, for example, marital difficulties, disagreement about child rearing; consideration of the teenager's position in the family, both chronologically and in terms of authority within the family system; evidence of sibling rivalry; turntaking skills within family; parents' rate of speech; cultural expectations; bilingualism and the parents and child's capabilities within mother tongue and English; peer group attitudes towards teenager and evidence of pressures, bullying or teasing are all considered.

It is not suggested that the areas outlined above are in any way exhaustive. They are essentially a product of the numerous interviews carried out over several years with this client group and individual clinicians may include other issues as applicable. The elements should not, of course, be considered in isolation, as each is interdependent upon the other. However, the relative importance of each element which presents in the overall picture of the young adult client should advise and influence the clinician in the focus, structure and chronicity of her plan for intervention. We present four case studies to illustrate this notion and to show how we have used this grid approach in our own management of these individual cases.

Case study

Errol was the 17-year-old only child of Turkish Cypriot parents who was referred to our clinic by his very concerned mother for assessment and treatment of, in his mother's words, 'his very severe stutter'. Errol presented at interview with his parents as a reluctant participant, who, by his own admission, was sceptical about the help that our service could offer him.

There was no evidence of family history of stuttering given by either parent at this stage. The stutter had developed from the age of 7 and had grown noticeably worse when the family returned to live in Cyprus when Errol was 10. The family had returned to live in England two years later, as they were unhappy in Cyprus, largely due to parental conflict with the extended family and a failure to integrate into the cultural system there. His general health was good with the usual childhood ailments, but no serious health problems.

During fluency assessment, Errol presented 4.5% stuttered words and an average speech rate of 139 words per minute and his stuttering behaviour was characterised by some word repetition and minimal blocking behaviour. There was little evidence of word avoidance, however, his eye-contact was very poor and his listening skills also appeared limited and there was evidence of situation avoidance. He had no other learning difficulties, indeed, he was doing very well at school, studying for four 'A' levels, however, he had a history of aggression towards his peers in his early adolescence.

Errol felt that he performed badly in certain social situations, including using the telephone, talking in front of large groups, asking questions of teachers, talking to girls and speaking to strangers. He felt that periods of more acute dysfluency were often preceded by him being asked questions in front of his peers; being asked questions requiring highly specific answers, e.g. in physics; when he was tired or angry. The consequences of the dysfluency were usually that he felt embarrassed, angry and 'useless'. He would avoid those situations for a short while following the episode of dysfluency, but would recognise that he should attempt them again, which he did, with variable success. He felt that he had some control over the stutter, but this was not consistent.

Errol had a limited range of friends, all male. He desired closer contact with members of the opposite sex within his social group, but he was not confident or sure how he should go about this as he was worried about being rejected and 'failing'.

Errol had very high self-expectations and high expectations of his parents. His father never measured up to the expectations Errol had of him, however, a fact which made his father seem 'weak' and 'useless' in Errol's eyes. Errol felt that his father was emotionally distant and he could not relate to him 'as a father or a man'. Errol had on two occasions attempted to instigate a physical fight with his father in recent months. The father had 'failed' to react physically, a fact which exacerbated Errol's anger and resentment towards him. Errol's relationship with his mother was intensely emotional, but ambivalent. He loved her very much but she was emotionally unpredictable and had severe mood swings. She would also hit her husband during their frequent rows and she admitted that she felt that he had failed her as a husband, in every sense, during most of their 17-year marriage. The parents had a poor sex life, mother felt that the rare sexual contact which did take place was always initiated by her and that there was little emotional rapport between them. Father presented as a quietly spoken man who clearly found it difficult to discuss his feelings or thoughts but expressed a desire to help his son however he could.

The family was financially secure and Errol had his own room in a large, comfortable house, where the family had lived for the last five years. Errol had a regular allowance of £50 per month, which he felt was adequate for his needs.

Upon completion of the parental and adolescent assessments it became clear that there were a number of complex, interdependent issues within the family dynamic, as well as considerable intra-personal factors specific to the boy himself, in terms of his capacities and his own belief systems, which we felt were likely to be contributing to the ostensibly mild, yet persistent stuttering behaviour.

Within the context of our grid we identified the following factors:

- Physiological: there was a relatively late onset of stuttering behaviour, which appeared to be exacerbated by the major life change of moving to Cyprus. The overt stuttering behaviour itself was mild but clearly affected the boy's own performance and motivation. Rate of speech was relatively high.
- Cognitive–emotional: Errol had high self-expectations, including being able to cure his stutter. He was afraid of failure in any context, indeed 'failure' was a derogatory term often used in the expression of his own belief system. His locus of control was ambivalent, for although he felt he could have some influence on life events, his problem-solving strategies in response to possible or actual failure were negligible. He had limited empathy for the feelings of others and this was intensified in his relationship with his father, whom he did not

understand. He was at the same time intensely attached to and frightened of his mother, who continued to play the dominant role in his life. He demonstrated aggression rather than assertion in his dealings with others and had a limited social network as a consequence.

- Behavioural: there were clear antecedents and consequences to the stuttering behaviour and it is significant that Errol was able to identify these in relationship to what appeared to be an overtly mild difficulty. The behaviour was somewhat adaptive across a range of situations, some of which were very problematic for him, others which were more straightforward. Errol did not possess a wide range of peer group relationships and this was a source of concern for him. His social communication skills were limited, he would often appear to be aggressive, verbally and physically, towards his parents. Although his academic performance was good, he was ambivalent about this and was adversely affected by any slip in performance.

- Environmental: the family circumstances were of key importance in this case. Whilst there were no financial or residential concerns, the family dynamics were clearly dysfunctional. Although Errol had his own room, his mother would often enter the room with little or no warning. She had found pornography in his room and, although she was not angry about this, she wished to discuss it with Errol in detail, which he found painful and embarrassing. Hence, he did not have an inviolable 'space of his own'. There were obvious problems in the relationships between each of the family members with one another. Errol felt the need for a relationship with his father, yet he resented him and his failure to provide this function. Mother had maintained an intensely jealous relationship with the boy and had isolated the father who could not fulfil her expectations as a husband.

The parental expectations of the boy were considerable. The mother expected the boy to be her emotional support in the absence of such support from the father. The father was at some level colluding with this arrangement by not asserting his own role either in relationship to his son or his wife. There were expectations of the boy to be a 'success', to be happy and to be fluent. He attended a high-achieving school where there was an emphasis on high academic performance. There were also significant issues in the extended family dynamic. There was conflict between the family and their extended family in Cyprus. The mother felt that there were expectations of all of them which they could not meet and this made her angry and resentful, particularly towards her mother in law who was the matriarch of the family. This attitude had also been adopted by Errol who felt that the extended family were ignorant and bigoted. Whilst the first language in the home was English, father's command of it was not as proficient as that of either mother or Errol. Turkish was also spoken at home on occasions.

Feedback to family

Whilst the information disclosed to the clinician from this case was of a highly sensitive and personal nature it was felt appropriate to feedback most of the issues identified above in a summarised form, in order that the family could understand the rationale behind the proposed intervention programme. In the event, the family concurred with the summary and were willing to accept the programme of intervention suggested.

Recommendations for intervention

To offer Errol a package of four individual therapy sessions, once per fortnight in the first instance, on a trial basis, to see whether he found it helpful. The focus of these sessions would initially be targeted towards:

- The physiology of the problem, i.e. the dysfluency itself, introducing fluency-enhancing strategies, such as slowing rate of speech and easy onset, as outlined in Chapter 4 of this book.
- Behavioural aspects of the dysfluency, including identification of difficult speaking situations, identification of antecedents and consequences of the behaviour, social communication skills, problem-solving strategies in relation to these situations and experimentation, practice and role play using video facilities, to gain feedback on performance and progress.

The focus of this initial programme of therapy was intentionally taken off the emotional–cognitive and environmental issues which were clearly contributing significantly to the problem. This was in an attempt to engage Errol into the therapeutic process. He was a wary young man, who had not attended the clinic on an entirely voluntary basis. Therefore, we felt we needed to concentrate, in the first instance, upon relatively non-emotive work, with a view to entering the deeper arena of his own emotions and attitudes at the appropriate juncture. In the event, this was the correct decision.

- That the parents should attend for counselling with a suitably qualified therapist in order to resolve some of their marital difficulties. The intention behind this was to attempt to alleviate some of the pressure from Errol and to focus the parents' communication on themselves.
- That Errol should take responsibility for looking after his own bedroom. He should make his own bed, put out dirty laundry in an appropriate place outside his own room on a regular basis and vacuum the room at reasonable intervals. The agreement with his mother was that she would not enter his room unless invited to do so by Errol. He, in turn, agreed that his mother could remind him to

carry out the domestic tasks if he was not carrying them out as agreed. In this way we secured a sanctuary for Errol, which he badly needed, in order to establish his first sense of separateness from his mother and her conflicts with his father.

• That Errol and his father should carry out a 'quality time' task together. This entailed a minimum of three sessions per week, of 10 minutes' duration which Errol and his father would spend together. The topic(s) during the 'quality time' should be non-emotive in content initially, focusing on a mutual recreational activity in the first instance. Progress with this task was to be recorded on homework sheets and monitored closely by the therapists working with the family. The purpose of this task was to attempt to re-open channels of communication between Errol and his father, initially at a simple level, in the hope that their relationship would begin to develop as they became more used to each others' company.

Update

It was anticipated that Errol would need gradual introduction to the process of disclosure of feelings and emotions surrounding his dysfluency, as this was so deeply embedded in his relationship with his parents. However, after the initial package of four sessions he volunteered to continue in therapy. Indeed, he requested that he should be able to increase the frequency of his sessions to once weekly. During the first therapy session it was made clear to him that therapy would have four major components: physiological; behavioural; cognitive–emotional, and environmental. He found this structure helpful in understanding the nature of his problem and the intervention proposed. Meanwhile, the parents have made considerable progress in resolving some of their own difficulties and have begun to communicate with each other in a more satisfactory manner. However, it was anticipated that Errol might find this re-alignment of his parents' relationship difficult to tolerate and understand. This became evident through a deterioration in his relationship with his mother as he became verbally and physically abusive towards her for a short period. Therapy at this stage was targeted towards encouraging him to verbalise his feelings of resentment and anxiety about this change in the family's status quo, facilitating more constructive problem-solving strategies in relation to the problem and, above all, ensuring that the lines of communication were kept open between Errol and his parents through regular joint family sessions.

Case study

'James and his family were referred to our clinic by his local speech and language therapist. At 17, he was the youngest of three boys in a stable household, with both parents living at home.'

'There was some history of stuttering within the extended family. James' maternal grandfather had a stutter as a child and it was occasionally apparent throughout his adult life, although it was never as severe a problem as that presented by James. The grandfather had died two years previously. James had enjoyed a very close relationship with him and had found it difficult to come to terms with his death.'

'James had demonstrated dysfluent behaviour from the age of 3. His parents had initially been advised to ignore the problem by their local GP, as he thought it was likely that the child would grow out of the problem. The dysfluency became progressively worse until, at the age of 8, James' parents requested speech and language therapy. James subsequently attended for therapy at a local level over a 2-year period, but the dysfluency proved resistant to intervention.'

'Typically, the pattern would be that James would attend an intensive therapy course for one week, which was targeted at teaching fluency-enhancing speech modification techniques. There would be an improvement in fluency immediately following these programmes but James then found it difficult to maintain this improvement.'

'His general health was excellent, although his parents did admit that he was prone to occasional, mysterious stomach aches during his primary school career, when he would miss school for one or two days at a time.'

'During assessment, James demonstrated a severe dysfluency problem. An average of 36% stuttered words was gained, with a speech rate of 98 words per minute. The dysfluency was typified by significant struggle behaviour associated with prolongations and part-word, whole-word and phrase repetitions.'

'He was doing well at a mixed sex, sixth form college, studying for four 'A' levels.'

'James had very poor self-image and esteem, focused largely around his stuttering behaviour. He wanted the stutter to be cured, for if this was achieved he felt that his life would be devoid of any problems and he would function just like any other lad of his age. As it was, he was 'frightened' of speaking to teachers, groups of people, relatives, strangers and, especially, members of the opposite sex. He felt that there was little he could do about his stutter, it was predictable in that it 'happens all the time'. However, James had no strategies for improving fluency or gaining any control over it.'

'He presented as a sensitive young man, with a clear sense of empathy for others and considered himself to be a good friend. His eye-contact was poor, although his listening skills were fair. He had a good range of friends, mainly male, of his own age or older, and enjoyed playing sports. However, he found it extremely difficult to talk about his own feelings to either friends or family and appeared to have a limited range of vocabulary in order to express his considerable state of distress with regard to his severe speech difficulty.'

'James had an acute fear of failure, as exemplified by a recent suicide attempt before referral. This had been precipitated because he had been required to work on the cash register of the food store where he held a part-time job. Hitherto, he had been stacking shelves, but now he was required to speak to customers directly and, of particular concern, to speak over a tannoy system where his voice could be heard throughout the store usually stuttering severely. He had endured eight weekends of this painful experience, without discussing it with the manager of the store, his colleagues or family. He had become so distressed that on the Friday prior to the ninth weekend, he had taken a relatively small overdose of aspirin and absconded from home. He was found by the police in the early hours of the following day and was admitted to hospital for emergency treatment. As a consequence of this experience, James was referred to a specialist unit for outpatient counselling with a psychologist. However, it was felt that James should be referred to a speech and language therapist as his problems were so bound up with the overt stuttering behaviour.'

'James could not identify particular antecedents of the dysfluency, but it had obvious consequences ranging from chronic situation avoidance, sense of failure, anger and frustration. The stutter was minimally adaptive across situations, although it did improve when he was talking to his brothers. It was usually poor with his parents.'

'There were no overt problems within the parental relationship. They had been happily married for 26 years, enjoyed each others' and their children's company and had a wide and varied social network of family and friends. Mother had been depressed around the time of her father's death and found it difficult to come to terms with the fact that he was no longer present as she had enjoyed a close relationship with him.'

'Both parents were highly anxious and bewildered by James' suicide attempt and very concerned that he might try it again. However, they had found it difficult to talk to James about the experience and it became clear that mother in particular found James' stutter embarrassing and distressing. She would often avoid eye-contact with him when he became dysfluent and would finish sentences for him or offer advice regarding how he might become more fluent. This annoyed James intensely, and he consequently found it very hard to talk to his mother about his situation.'

'Father saw himself as being similar in nature to James (a view James shared), in that he was a shy man, who found it difficult to talk about emotional issues and tended to keep things 'bottled up'.'

'Both parents were relatively rapid speakers who were observed to talk across each other. James' brothers were aged 20 and 23, respectively. They shared a close relationship with James, he was definitely the 'younger brother'; they were protective of him and tended to speak for him in social situations. James was popular at college, considered to be quiet and diligent by his teachers who were unaware of his recent emotional crisis.'

'James had his own room in a comfortable, spacious house and received a regular allowance from his parents, since leaving the part-time job he had held previously.'

The following issues were identified within the context of the grid:

- Physiological factors: there was a family history of stuttering on the maternal side of the family. There was also an early developmental onset and secondary, advanced stuttering characteristics were evident. Whereas general health was good, the inexplicable stomach aches as a child were likely to be psychosomatic in nature, possibly indicating early situation avoidance. The stuttering behaviour was severe in nature across a range of situations. Speech was characterised by relatively rapid bursts of speech interspersed with severe blocks and struggle behaviour, therefore speech rate was also considered an issue which needed to be addressed.

- Cognitive–emotional: James had very poor self-image and esteem and had very limited problem-solving strategies. This was exacerbated by an inability to express his feelings and emotions to others, thus leading to the extreme action of the suicide attempt, which was a cry for help. James reported later that he never wished to actually kill himself. Whilst James appeared to be quite empathic and considered himself a good friend, this was not supported by his reluctance to enter into dialogue regarding issues of an emotional nature. James was dependent upon his family, especially his older brothers, for many things and this system had become a habit within the family. He loved his parents very much, but felt that they did not understand the severity of his speech problem and its implications for his life. The effects of his grandfather's death upon James had been underestimated, it was felt that he had not grieved adequately for his loss and this was not openly discussed in the family.

- Behavioural: there was a pressing need for James to understand more clearly the antecedents to the stuttering behaviour and more explicit disclosure of the consequences was also required. It appeared initially that his stutter was minimally adaptive. However, more investigation of the reality of this situation was necessary in order to understand the problem. James had a wide ranging social network, but he was not using his close friends as emotional support, even at a time of extreme crisis. He had attempted suicide, but as yet, had proven resistant to intimate disclosure of the motivations underlying the action.

- Environmental: the family unit was stable, loving and caring towards each of its members, including James. There were some parental expectations of James in relationship to academic performance, as he was perceived as a bright boy. However, one of his older brothers was not a high achiever in school and the parents had accepted this unequivocally. Their stated philosophy was 'You can only do your best'. The parents' marriage was secure and they openly discussed their worries and concerns with each other, although not very often with their sons. Turntaking within conversations was also an issue which needed addressing, as family members often interrupted each other, with mother's rapid rate of speech also being an added dimension to this problem.

Feedback to parents

The grid was used to feedback the issues outlined above to the parents and James, following the diagnostic interview. They reported that they had found the structure very helpful in understanding more clearly the context of the stutter and how the family dynamics played such an important part in the problem. This deeper insight was to prove critical in the success of the intervention programme proposed for James and his family.

Recommendations for intervention

That James should attend for an initial package of six, once-weekly, therapy sessions. The initial focus of these sessions would be to gain a clearer understanding of the physiological and behavioural components of the stuttering behaviour by:

- Exploring effective speech modification techniques with James, such as easy onset, flowing speech and soft contacts.
- Identifying a hierarchy of difficult speaking situations, by use of the PQRST assessment of attitudes (Mulhall, 1977).
- To identify antecedents and consequences of stuttering behaviour and to plan a behavioural programme of assignments to begin to facilitate change in these in order to enhance fluency.
- To teach and practise effective social communication skills, including the importance of eye-contact, observation skills and problem-solving skills.
- To explore the emotions surrounding the dysfluency with James on an individual basis, once a relationship of trust had been established between him and the therapist.
- To facilitate disclosure by encouraging him to retell the story of his suicide attempt on a structured chronological basis. That is, to go through the antecedents, stage by stage, encouraging him to express his feelings at each stage leading up to the final action.
- To discuss the death of his grandfather in a similar, stage by stage, fashion to allow James to complete the grieving process.
- To teach James specific problem-solving techniques. To review the exploration of emotions as outlined above and encourage James to apply an appropriate problem-solving strategy to this situation. That is, 'What could I have done differently and when?'. To continue to encourage James to apply such techniques to other problems in his life, both speech and non-speech related, as they occur and to bring these to the therapy sessions for exploration with the therapist.
- To set up a 'quality time' task between James and his mother and, separately, with James and his father, three times a week each for a minimum of 5 minutes, the emphasis being placed on the parents slowing their own rate of speech and also allowing James to finish what he had to say. This was practised in the clinic first to ensure that

the parents and James had understood that task.

At the end of the 6-week package of sessions to hold a family review to evaluate progress to date and the way forward. Agreement was reached with James, before this meeting, upon the issues which could be divulged to his parents, in addition to his proposals for change in their management strategies.

Update

Although James made good progress in establishing better fluency, he found the process of disclosure very difficult during the later therapy sessions. Indeed, he needed a great deal of help in order to find the vocabulary which adequately expressed his feelings about his experiences. He benefited from the visual presentation of problem-solving strategies, however, and he found the structured nature of these exercises actually helped him to organise his thoughts about the generalised sense of pain he felt about his suicide attempt, his grandfather's death and his stutter. In this way, he was able to become more specific and explicit about his problems and we began to move him towards a clearer perspective concerning his dysfluency and its place in his world. As his understanding of the complexity of the problem increased, his avoidance strategies decreased and his confidence in social situations grew. He continues to experience considerable fluency difficulties, however, the problem is increasingly adaptive and James feels a more tangible sense of control.

His parents have carried out their tasks diligently and have maintained regular contact with the therapist. James continues in individual therapy, on a 6-week package basis, with an inbuilt schedule of review.

Case study

'Lisa was a 16-year-old only child. She lived in a comfortable home, with her own room, with both her parents and the decision to refer her to our centre had been made by the family as a whole.'

'There was no family history of stuttering. Lisa had first started having problems with her fluency from the age of 4 and, from the age of 8, there was an extensive history of intervention from speech and language therapists and psychologists. Although her general health was excellent, she was very concerned that she might have to give up her contact lenses because of chronic conjunctivitis.'

'She demonstrated a severe dysfluency with an average of 42% stuttered words and a speech rate of 78 words per minute. Her dysfluency was characterised by severe blocks at bilabial, alveolar and pharyngeal level, with associated struggle and voice onset problems. Her eye-contact during dysfluency oscillated from a constant stare to total absence. Other concomitant features included significant evidence of word avoidance and situational avoidance, hand flapping and head shaking. Lisa felt that she lacked any control over her stutter and that it was entirely unpredictable.'

'This sense of lack of control seemed to pervade many other areas of her life, including relationships with her peers. She had poor self-image, feeling that she was unattractive and stupid. At that time she was studying for 10 GCSE's at a mixed sex, local comprehensive and her parents report was that she was, in fact, one of the brightest pupils in her year.'

'Lisa had great empathy for others and was involved in a number of philanthropic campaigns and felt passionately for the 'underdog'. She viewed herself as the victim of circumstances, stating that she felt that her stutter was 'unfair'.'

'Lisa had a stormy relationship with her mother, they argued frequently, often about Lisa's stutter and the fact that she was dependent upon her parents to carry out the 'simplest tasks' such as making telephone calls. Her mother's view was that if only Lisa tried harder to overcome her stutter she would conquer it. Lisa felt that her mother did not understand her.'

'Lisa had a close relationship with her father, who spent long periods away from home on business trips. Father admitted to a feeling of helplessness with regard to Lisa's dysfluency, becoming tearful during the parental interview when questioned about it.'

'Lisa demonstrated minimal problem-solving strategies and an overt fear of failure and avoidance of a wide range of social situations. Lisa was unable to identify the antecedents to her stuttering behaviour and, indeed, could not give an objective analysis of the actual behaviour at all. She felt that it was severe across most situations, although it was significantly better with her best female friend, to whom she was very close and other peers with whom she was familiar. She was subsequently able to identify specific situations when her speech became markedly worse.'

'Lisa had a fair range of peer group relationships, of both sexes and previously had had a regular boyfriend for about six months. Although popular with girls and boys Lisa felt that she might lose her friends if they thought she appeared 'stupid'. She presented as a physically attractive young woman.'

'During the parental interview, it became apparent that there were significant difficulties within the marriage. There was considerable tension between the two parents during the interview, they argued openly regarding Lisa and her speech problem as well as other issues within the family, including the state of their own relationship. Lisa had been a result of an unplanned pregnancy. It subsequently transpired that the mother was conducting an extra-marital affair of which the father was at that stage unaware. Mother expressed considerable anger towards Lisa, her husband and the professionals who had been unable to 'cure' her daughter's problem in the past.'

'Both parents' rates of speech were rapid, both were voluble personalities and both expressed deep scepticism about the need for them to be involved in what was, after all, their daughter's problem.'

'There was limited contact between Lisa and her extended family, although she felt close to her maternal grandparents.'

'Lisa did not receive a regular allowance, approaching her parents when she wanted to purchase clothes, make up and other sundry items. She was not at all happy with this situation and was attempting to get a part-time job.'

Upon completion of the diagnostic interview the following issues were extrapolated from the information gained:

- Physiological factors: there was an early developmental onset of dysfluency which had been unresponsive to previous intervention. The dysfluency was advanced, with secondary characteristics, including situation avoidance and severe struggle.
- Cognitive–emotional: low self-esteem and self-image were apparent. Very limited sense of control over the problem with ambivalent self-expectations—wanting to achieve, yet feeling it was impossible. Highly empathic, possibly as a result of own feelings of victimisation and unhappiness. Dysfunctional relationship with mother over many years. Unresolved resentment and bitterness expressed on both sides. Relationship with father close but sporadic. Limited problem-solving skills and disabling fear of failure. No financial independence or experience of budgeting for self.
- Behavioural: antecedents to the stuttering behaviour were unclear and required further investigation. Consequences were significant, resulting in embarrassment, distress and future avoidance strategies. The stutter was minimally adaptive, although this had not been fully explored and Lisa did not have any real sense of prediction or control over the dysfluency. Lisa had a good, range of supportive friends.
- Environmental: Lisa had her own room for which she was responsible domestically. Significant parent–child conflict and parent–parent conflict. Lisa's stutter had become the focus for the family's frustration and anger, deflecting attention away from the other significant problems within the family dynamic. Therefore, at an unconscious level, the stutter was serving a purpose in keeping the family together. How likely was it therefore, that the problem would respond to intervention, whilst those other issues remained unresolved? Parents' rapid rate of speech and models of turntaking needed addressing. Parental expectations were high, both academically and in terms of resolution of the severe, chronic dysfluency problem.

Recommendations for intervention

Lisa should initially have six individual, once weekly, therapy sessions focused on:

- Improvement of fluency through fluency-enhancing techniques, including: flowing speech; easy onset and soft contacts, and breathing and relaxation.
- Behavioural aspects of the problem, including identification of

antecedents and situations of difficulty, social communication skills
training with role rehearsal, role play and experiential learning
featured within the intervention.

- That Lisa should attend a 2-week intensive therapy course for young
  adults, to be held within the next 3 months (the outline of this course
  is provided in Chapter 5).
- That the parents should be referred to an appropriately qualified
  therapist or marriage guidance counsellor in order to attempt to
  resolve some of their own conflicts and alleviate some of the pressure
  upon Lisa.
- To establish separate 'quality time' tasks between Lisa and each
  parent for a minimum of 5 minutes, three times per week. There
  were to be no arguments during these sessions, and if this seemed
  unavoidable, the session was to be terminated immediately and post-
  poned. This was to be monitored closely by the therapist via homework sheets completed by each parent and Lisa.
- Lisa was to receive a regular allowance every month which was nego-
  tiated with the parents and Lisa. She was to be responsible for
  budgeting this allowance. In this way we began to develop the notion
  of Lisa's independence from her parents in order to improve her self-
  esteem and confidence in her own abilities.

Update

In the event, Lisa's parents separated with the intention of divorce
following marriage guidance sessions where they decided that their
marital problems were unlikely to resolve. Despite a significant deterioration in fluency, Lisa persisted with her therapy sessions after her
parent's separation. Following the initial phase of fluency enhancement
and behavioural change, the therapy progressed towards exploration of
the emotional and cognitive aspects of her stutter. She attended the
intensive course recommended and achieved considerable improvement in her fluency, independence, problem-solving and social skills
which continue to develop and increase.

Lisa completed and passed her three 'A' levels, her driving test and
she is doing well in her first job. She is seeking her own flat to share with
a friend and her relationship with both parents is, in her opinion, more
stable. Lisa continues to attend for individual sessions on a review only
basis.

Case study

'John was 15 when he was referred to our clinic by his parents. They were
concerned about his stutter as he wished to join the Air Force and become a
pilot upon leaving school. John was keen to attend the centre for treatment
as he felt that speech and language therapy might help him to overcome the

problem before he applied to join the armed forces. He was the eldest of two boys both living at home. His younger brother was 12 and had moderate learning difficulties.'

'John's mother had also stuttered as a child, she was very occasionally dysfluent and had numerous strategies for overcoming the behaviour.'

'John's own dysfluency had first become apparent at the age of 5 when he changed schools following the family's move from Scotland to southern England. At that time, John had been teased considerably by his new peers about his accent.'

'Apart from the removal of his appendix at the age of 11, his general health was very good.'

'Upon assessment, John's dysfluency was observed to be in the mild range, with an average of 3.5% stuttered words and a speech rate of 142 words per minute. His dysfluency was characterised by some hesitations, part-word and whole-word repetitions with some word avoidance reported although not obvious during assessment. There was some evidence of dyslexia, his writing was difficult to read and disorganised, although the content was appropriate. He had had some extra tuition at school during his primary years. However, he was doing quite well now but said that he hated French as he 'did not get on with the teacher'.'

'John did not see his stutter as a major obstacle in his life. He was a confident, extrovert young man who expected to do well in his exams at school and was determined to achieve his career ambitions. He was popular at school, being captain of the rugby team and enjoying a good relationship with his peers and most of his teachers. He often spent time away from his family during trips away with the Junior Air Corps which he enjoyed immensely. He found the notion of failure 'unacceptable', and did not wish to contemplate any alternatives to his overabiding ambitions to do well at school and become a pilot. Indeed, he could foresee no obstacles in the way of his achieving his career plans.'

'John had some insight into the antecedents of the stuttering problem, which he identified as feelings of stress or pressure, attempting to enter into conversations which were already underway, answering questions which required specific answers, giving orders, e.g. when teamleading in Air Corps exercises and speaking on the telephone. The consequences were mainly identified as increased tension, embarrassment, annoyance at self and a slight worsening of the problem for a brief period. However, he did not avoid situations—this would be 'weak' in his view and he considered that the speech could be controlled eventually.'

'The family lived in a small, three-bedroomed house. John shared a room with his brother and the two argued frequently. The parents had a stable, loving marriage of 22 years. They had expectations of John to do well at school and, although they realised that he did not find school work easy, he had the self-discipline and determination to succeed which they hoped would allow him to do well. They felt that his younger brother was very demanding of their time and felt guilty about this on John's account. John felt a strong, protective attachment to his brother but he was frustrated with his unpredictable behaviour and interference with his possessions.'

'The parents' rate of speech was relatively rapid and turntaking was an issue at home as they admitted that they often interrupted John when he was talking to them.'

'The school's expectations were generally felt to be fair, but there had recently been some conflict with the French teacher who had made John stand up and read in front of the class. She had stopped him when he had stuttered and asked him why he was doing it. He had lost his temper and run from the class. His classmates had boycotted the rest of the class in response to her behaviour and as a consequence she had placed him on detention. He felt that her behaviour had been unreasonable. The parents had requested a meeting with the teacher, but had been unable to persuade her to manage John differently.'

'John had a part-time job as a paper-delivery boy.'

The issues extrapolated from this case history were as follows:

- Physiological: there was a significant family history of stuttering behaviour, mother describing herself as a 'stutterer'. There had been a relatively early onset of the behaviour possibly exacerbated by move from Scotland, and the short-term problems in peer integration. Whilst the stuttering behaviour itself was within the mild range, the speech rate was relatively rapid and sometimes affected intelligibility. There was evidence of other learning difficulties and these would need further exploration although it appeared that John had developed good compensatory strategies.
- Cognitive–emotional: John had a positive self-image with ambivalent feelings towards the stuttering behaviour which he considered an 'irritation'. He was an assertive boy, who enjoyed social contact with his peers. However, he often appeared to talk at length, at the cost of listening to what was being said to him. On occasions he admitted that he had hurt the feelings of friends, particularly girls, by being too forthright in his views and his tendency to tell others what to do about their problems. He liked to be in control, or in charge of situations and was proud of his ability to make decisions quickly and act upon them. Unfortunately, he had on occasion made the wrong decision and suffered the consequences. Hence, he needed the opportunity to develop his social skills, including observation, listening, turntaking, negotiation and problem-solving.
- Behavioural: there was a need for social skills training, as identified above. The stuttering behaviour was adaptive, but John needed to develop deeper insights into antecedents and consequences. Good range of peer relationships, however, perhaps over dominant? Reasonable academic performance, but this required a dedicated effort on John's part—what would happen if he failed to achieve?
- Environmental: stable family background. However, a need for more positive turntaking and listening skills within family dynamic. Need for own room as soon as possible to establish independence from younger brother; both need own sense of space. Opportunity for

own quality time with parents. Parental rate of speech. Expectations/management issues within school which need to be addressed.

Feedback to family

All of the issues above were discussed openly with the parents and John. Whereas John had some initial difficulties accepting the need for social skills training, he agreed to 'try it out' on the basis proposed in the intervention plan, which was as follows.

That John should attend a 2-week intensive course, focusing on the communication skills approach within the next 3 months.

In the intervening period a 'quality time' task was set up between each parent and John. The focus of these sessions was to:

- Attempt to slow down the rate of speech.
- Make a more conscious attempt to take turns and to keep interruptions to a minimum. Both of these strategies were practised within the clinic setting.
- Allow John and his parents to plan more frequent quality time together and to plan family activities.
- Referral on to a specialist in dyslexia to assess any residual difficulties and develop strategies which would be helpful to John.
- That John should move into the spare bedroom in the house and establish his own space. He would be responsible for the general domestic upkeep of his room.
- Following John's attendance on the intensive course, the therapist would arrange a visit to the school in order to run a training session for the teachers within the school and devise a management programme with those teachers who had direct contact with John.

Update

John attended the 2-week intensive course as recommended. He progressed extremely well, his level of fluency stabilised and he made a noticeable improvement in his awareness and use of social communication skills. His parents found the task of slowing their own speech down very difficult to put into practice, indeed, initially they avoided the task. The therapist was required to recall them into the centre and to practise the task with them again as well as investigating their own anxieties about it. This done, they carried out their homework more diligently, however, it remained a problem for them for some time. John was keen to help his parents carry out their task effectively, however, and assumed a monitoring role for them.

Assessment by a dyslexia specialist identified some minimal higher-level language problems, associated with word retrieval and some strategies were suggested.

A training session was run at the school which proved to be very productive. Basic behavioural management strategies were agreed and implemented by teaching staff and these were, in fact, extended to other pupils within the school who stuttered. These included negotiating with John a system where he could indicate to a teacher that he felt able to read in front of the class; allowing him to continue reading until he had finished a passage without interruption; overt, positive reinforcement when he had completed a speaking task; paired speaking activities with a fluent peer and a 5-minute individual session on a periodic basis with a class teacher to discuss the stutter openly. John's performance in French is steadily improving.

Summary

We have presented these case studies in the hope that they illustrate our own approach to planning appropriate interventions in response to the wealth of information to be gathered from the diagnostic interview process. We have found the structure of our grid invaluable in clarifying the contributory factors and how these relate to one another as well as providing a framework within which we can summarise the key issues of the stuttering problem.

To treat the problem in isolation, we believe, is to ignore its complexity and to underestimate its effects on the adolescent who stutters. We do not claim that this is an easy task for any clinician. However, with the application of our professional skills, we believe that positive change can be achieved for young adults, their families and carers. The key skills being active listening, flexibility, imagination and creativity in dealing with the broad range of issues which will arise from the process of family based assessment.

In subsequent chapters we expand our approach to the therapeutic process by describing the content of the interventions themselves; how we rationalise them, give them structure and apply them within a group intensive framework. This is not intended as a recipe for therapy, rather as examples from which speech and language clinicians might draw inspiration for adoption, modification or adaptation to their own circumstances and their own clients.

Chapter 4
Communication Skills Approach

This chapter will describe our communication skills approach to therapy with the rationale for each of the interdependent components. The practical application of these is fully described in the following chapter.

This therapeutic approach is concerned with helping the person who stutters to make changes in a number of areas concerning communication skills and his perception of both himself and others. Sheehan (1970) emphasised that stuttering occurs in communicative situations where others are present—'it takes two to stutter'. He described stuttering as a disorder of 'Interpersonal self-presentation, occurring in a social context'.

A substantial part of our lives is spent interacting with other people, and the success or failure of these encounters can profoundly influence our development as individuals. By adolescence, the person who stutters is likely to have experienced many failures in communication. He will have developed a number of complex strategies for dealing with certain problematic situations and new difficulties will emerge daily which will have to be incorporated into therapy.

The person who stutters frequently attributes all his problems to the stuttering behaviour, thus making it the focal point in his life.

Self-concepts and relationships

The establishment of social relationships within the family and later outside the family is central to healthy, adaptive functioning (Rustin and Kuhr, 1989). Communication is of the utmost importance in establishing and maintaining relationships. If a child's verbal communication skill is restricted, opportunities to participate in satisfying interactions and form good relationships are reduced. It has been shown repeatedly that the perception of 'similarity' is important from early childhood to early adolescence (Rubin and Ross, 1982). The individual who is significantly different from his peer group will be perceived as less attractive and therefore his chances of normal social development will be diminished.

A feeling of helplessness or hopelessness may develop from repeated social failures and result in substantial social anxiety as well as depression.

In order to enhance the quantity and quality of social interactions in children and adults who stutter, we need to conceptualise interpersonal failures as being founded in the developmental experiences of each individual.

The behavioural approach alone is insufficient when considering the complexities of social interactions. Cognitive and affective aspects need to be included in any programme of behavioural change.

The role of cognitions, affective state and attitudes in social difficulties is widely acknowledged (Nichols, 1974). Beliefs about oneself, expectations of failure, anxiety and apprehension affect the individual's general level of motivation.

Motivation is a common theme when discussing therapeutic progress for clients. It is not that motivation is lacking, but that the overwhelming sense of probable failure may reduce drive. For the person who stutters to feel in control, he will need to understand his own thought processes and improve problem-solving abilities.

Rustin and Kuhr (1989) suggest that a number of skills are necessary in order to carry out the sophisticated interdependent interactions required in communication. These include:

• Viewing one's strengths realistically.
• Recognising and labelling one's emotions in relation to external events.
• Being empathic, i.e. aware of the feelings of others which would include the interpretation of verbal and non-verbal communication.

Rustin and Kuhr (1989) suggest that use of a cognitive–behavioural approach allows a progression from a 'more concrete level to a more abstract level and thus training focuses more on the process of interaction'. Cognitive–behaviour therapy explores higher level aspects of affect, including negative beliefs, unrealistic expectations and faulty attributions. Therapy aims to help the client to understand the emotions and consequent behaviours which are involved in social interaction, from both his own standpoint and those of other people. Therapy enables the client to explore the consequences of his own actions and the possibilities for change. Thus, the client is enabled to take personal responsibility for his own development by actively construing alternative strategies, developing hypotheses about the outcomes of these strategies and being given the opportunity to test these out.

The client becomes an active member of a therapeutic partnership with the implicit gains of self-monitoring, self-evaluation and self-reinforcement. These skills are essential to the transfer and maintenance of therapeutic gains.

As we have seen in the previous chapter, the necessity to tailor the therapy to the individual's needs is fundamental. To create a uniform treatment package, which is applied in a standard way to a group of clients who stutter, is to miss the essential nature of the problem—its individuality. Some dysfluency is found in otherwise healthy and psychologically stable adolescents; other cases of dysfluency may be associated with severe social, emotional or learning difficulties. In all instances the breadth and specific content of therapy needs to be unique to the individual.

Components of the communication skills therapy

The communication skills approach can be divided into six components. Although each is discussed individually, they are interdependent.

This treatment approach may be used successfully with groups or individuals on both intensive and non-intensive schedules. It maintains its flexibility throughout the client's progress. Therefore changes occurring as a result of therapy, or new factors emerging during therapy, can be accounted for to achieve the best possible outcome.

Each component has a cognitive and behavioural aspect which will be described and discussed. The therapy programme in the next chapter will elaborate the practical application of these components.

The six components of the communication skills approach are:

1. Fluency control.
2. Relaxation.
3. Social skills.
4. Problem-solving.
5. Negotiation.
6. Environmental factors.

In addition, the following assumptions may influence both client and clinician and need to be taken into account when designing the therapy programme. Omitting them would be to neglect important elements in the maintenance of stuttering:

- The underlying causes of stuttering remain of deep interest to the client and the clinician but therapy addresses those factors which are relevant to the 'here and now' of the client's life.
- The longer the adolescent has been stuttering the less chance he has of outgrowing the problem, therefore the clinician should not collude by promoting or allowing false hopes of cure for the client or the family.
- Most clients are able to predict, to some degree, the likelihood of

stuttering (i.e. the antecedents), for example, on specific words, in certain situations, or with particular people.
* Many clients associate moments of stuttering with feelings of anxiety, tension, loss of control, loss of confidence, and attribute these feelings to either the cause or the result of stuttering.
* Most clients have a fundamental belief that if only their speech problem could be 'cured' all other problems would be resolved.

Fluency control

Debate has continued through two decades as to whether stuttering should be shaped towards fluency, or modified towards more normal dysfluency (Peters and Guitar, 1991). Many clinicians are currently combining both the fluency-shaping and stuttering modification approaches in their programmes, with the focus on 'speech change' still the main emphasis in most programmes. Our approach views fluency control as one aspect of therapy, with equal weight being given to the other five components (relaxation, social skills, problem-solving, negotiation and environmental factors).

Frequently, clients state their desire to acquire normal fluency skills and share a belief with their parents that an improvement in their schoolwork, behaviour, attitudes and social life would be the result. Experimenting with fluency control techniques helps the person who stutters to adopt more realistic expectations of therapy. The more the client understands about his stuttering, the greater his chance of modifying the problem. It is our belief that the client should be encouraged to 'own' the stuttering. As long as a client has a concept of the stuttering coming 'out of the blue', 'something that just happens with no rhyme or reason', there can be no possibility of gaining control.

There are four stages within the fluency control component. Clients will need to understand all sections in order to use speech modification strategies effectively.

Stage 1: normal speech production

Few clients have a clear concept of how we produce speech. Like walking, 'you just get up and do it!'. It is necessary for the client to understand normal speech and language production in order to modify his own incorrect speech patterns. Thus, the role of breathing, voicing and articulation and their importance in the sequence of producing sounds, words and messages is discussed.

Stage 2: stuttering

Although there is no common definition for stuttering, we have found the following descriptive labels useful:

- Part-word repetitions, e.g. b.b.b.baby.
- Whole-word repetitions, e.g. but, but, but, but.
- Prolongations, e.g. ssssssseven.
- Struggle—where there are signs of physical tension.
- Silent blocks—these can be at any level of the vocal tract, but would indicate a complete cessation of sound.
- Associated behaviours, e.g. circumlocutions, avoidances, use of starters (e.g. 'actually', 'as a matter of fact'), or fillers (e.g. ums, ers, ahs, or other inappropriate words).

Brainstorming techniques (see p. 81) may be used to identify the general features of stuttering using the terminology described above.

In addition to these *measurable* aspects to stuttering, the more emotional components are discussed. These concern the feelings and emotions which are central to the stuttering problem. Indeed, a client is often able to identify the associated emotions clearly whilst being unable to describe the physical manifestations of his stuttering.

Sheehan (1970) uses the analogy of the stuttering iceberg to illustrate the overt aspects of speech dysfluency (the visible one-third of the iceberg) which are underpinned by the covert psychological aspects (the hidden two-thirds of the iceberg).

There are many stereotypes concerning stuttering and at this stage it is a useful exercise to explore the client's understanding of these, both from his own experience and his view of the perceptions of other people.

Stage 3: personal stuttering characteristics

At this stage, the clinician's theoretical standpoint is helpful in guiding the therapy process, but the client will need to feel that his personal theory of stuttering is valid and will be carefully explored. The client can then confirm or re-evaluate his original theory.

Linked to the notion of 'to put something right, you must know what has gone wrong', is the development of the individual's ability to recognise his own stuttering manifestations. This is consistent with many other treatment approaches which were embedded in the work of Van Riper (1982). The aim is therefore twofold:

1. For the client to understand the actual stuttering.
2. To desensitise the client by observing his own stuttering and thus, take 'ownership' of the problem.

This relates to the discussion on locus of control (see pages 12; 30). The client, by identifying and discussing the stuttering, is encouraged to assume a more internal locus of control, that is, he will be able to take more responsibility for the stutter. Although the actual moments of stuttering can be examined and explored, it is important to address the issues that relate to those behaviours which result from the stuttering: avoidances, concomitant movements, circumlocutions and extra strategies, such as speaking on residual air.

At the cognitive level, the client is enabled to understand what he is actually doing during stuttering and the additional features which are also part of the problem. The client is thus given the necessary tools to discuss, describe, dispute and contribute towards a mutual understanding.

A simple illustration of this would be the client who believes that all words beginning with /k/ are impossible. By analysing a tape-recorded sample it becomes apparent that this is not entirely accurate. A more complex example is the client who considers that every one else is totally fluent. Here, observations of normally non-fluent speakers through the use of videotaped samples demonstrates the fluency continuum. Alternatively, many clients maintain a theory that only people who stutter avoid using the telephone. An 'opinion poll' amongst friends and relatives will reveal that this is not necessarily the case. The aim with exercises like this is to broaden the client's perspective on stuttering.

Stage 4: fluency control

At this stage, the client and therapist examine those parameters of speech which need to be varied to promote improved fluency skills. The objective is to change as little as possible of the client's spontaneous speech while giving the feeling of greater speech control. The changes have to be 'user friendly'. Evidence is available from a variety of efficacy studies that the 'technical fluency' produced by many of the stuttering programmes does not transfer into the client's real world.

Perkins (1979) suggested that three conditions must be met before the clinician can expect a client to employ a speech modification technique:

1. Speech must sound normally expressive for the person concerned.
2. The skills for attaining fluency must be under voluntary control. It should be possible to describe these skills explicitly.
3. These skills should not be apparent when used.

Starkweather (1993) suggests that 'natural sounding speech is an appropriate therapeutic goal, but that the problem is broader than naturalness'. It is his opinion that 'fluent speech is simply speech that requires the least amount of motoric, linguistic, emotional and/or cognitive *effort* to produce'.

However, Gregory (1993) feels strongly that it is not inappropriate for a speaker to learn to monitor his own speech. Most effective professional speakers do just that, so that it is not unrealistic to ask a person who stutters to take extra care with his speech in certain circumstances. However, our aim of least difference from normal speech production, plus greater awareness of the factors which facilitate fluency, will enable the client to help himself more effectively.

The parameters that we identify as the fluency factors are:

- Rate control.
- Easy onsets.
- Flow of speech.
- Breath control.
- Soft contacts.

Rate Control

Although a number of authors define normal rates of speech, we consider that rate control implies the ability to modify the individual's natural speaking rate at will. A 17-year-old client suggested that stuttering was like driving a car, as you approach a difficult corner it is important to stay in control by changing gear and taking it carefully, once on the straight, the driver can then increase his speed. The person who stutters should learn to slow down his normal rate when approaching a problem word and, as he feels more in control ('on the straight') he can afford to go at his more natural rate. The skill is in learning to pace oneself.

Easy onsets

This describes a gentle or light contact of the articulators at the beginning of each new phrase. The first sound only of an utterance is said lightly and more slowly than normal ('slow motion'). Place and manner should remain as near normal as possible to maintain clarity. There can be a tendency for the affrication of plosives but this must be kept to the minimum.

Flow of speech

This refers to the feeling of continuous movement of the articulators during the utterance.

Breath control

Regulated breathing pattern should be used while avoiding overbreathing. Speaking on the egressive air stream with the concept of having 'enough' air without using residual airflow.

Soft contacts

All or some of the consonant sounds within a word are practised using a lighter contact point between articulators, principally on plosive sounds. Again, maintaining the place and manner of normal articulation as far as possible to obtain smooth movements of the articulators without slurring or omitting sounds.

Only clients at the moderate to severe end of the stuttering continuum would need to incorporate all fluency factors. For some clients, rate control would be sufficient, whereas others would find rate control plus easy onsets hold the key to improved fluency. Probably the most common combination at the beginning of therapy is rate control, easy onsets, flow and awareness of breath control. As therapy continues, dependence on some of the fluency factors decreases as the feeling of control develops.

The goal is to 'demystify' speech production by experiencing the exercises as if the client is improving a physical coordination skill. Despite the current debate concerning 'sub-clinical' stuttering and the controversy surrounding the normalcy of the fluent speech of those who stutter (Lees, in press), many clients report that they have some natural fluency. Our intention is to confirm conceptually that they can purposefully access this feeling of more control by practising in graded stages. The exercises, as with any behavioural programme, would commence at the easiest level. The self-monitoring of speech and the modification of targeted fluency factors are introduced in situations where there is least anticipation of a problem or, if possible, where there is no feeling of apprehension at all. Thus, the client initially becomes skilled at monitoring and changing elements of the speech production in situations of maximum control. Many clients observe that they find it impossible to include speech modification strategies in difficult situations, and at the same time identify this as their main aim in therapy. The introduction and practice of fluency factors in the easy situations with the client will ascertain:

• Whether the client can self-monitor.
• Whether the client can make the changes.

If these are not possible, then there would be no point in trying to attempt changes during speech situations identified as difficult. This aspect of the therapy is then reappraised with the client to consider the value of speech control methods at this stage. The partnership between client and therapist continuously deals with the 'why, what, where and how' questions, as well as the 'what if ...' and 'buts'. It may be that the client's expectations of therapy will need to be re-evaluated.

It is our view that part of the process of therapy is in both the client's and the parents' understanding that speech control is not necessarily the answer to all the problems of the adolescent who stutters. This allows those concerned to look at the wider issues involved in an atmosphere of shared understanding which, in turn, helps the client to take responsibility for his own fluency.

Relaxation

Relaxation training is widely used within the speech and language therapy field. Many alternative therapies also have physiological and mental relaxation as their focus for improved life skills. The state of relaxation is incompatible with feelings of fear, anger and anxiety. An increased awareness of the physiological manifestations of tension and ability to modify some aspects through relaxation training gives the client another dimension in the management of the stuttering problem. Again, it is not the whole answer but one of the component parts. Many clients focus on tension as their main difficulty, and this is compounded by the helpful advice liberally offered to most people who stutter, 'Just relax, calm down', etc. As one client explained '*I had tried to relax till I was blue in the face*'.

The purpose of relaxation is to give the client the ability to think of alternative ways of managing their physiological reactions in the context of their communication problem. It is, as with all our treatment strategies, critical to success that the client understands the concept of relaxation and this should be carefully explained before relaxation *per se* is taught.

Jacobson (1938) originated a relaxation technique in which patients are taught by alternately tensing and relaxing groups of muscles and being made aware of the differences between the sensation of tension and relaxation. It is common for clients to feel ill at ease during the first relaxation session but they should be encouraged to persevere. It takes a number of sessions before the skill is acquired.

Mitchell (1988) devised a relaxation regime which is physiologically based. The philosophy of this method is that conscious awareness of states of tension is provided by feedback from joints and skin, not muscles and tendons. Therefore, conscious relaxation is brought about by adjusting body posture. The instructions are simple and clear.

Social skills

Rustin and Kuhr (1989) found that deficits exist in the social skills repertoire of adults who stutter which contribute to their difficulties in maintaining long-term fluency. Rustin (1984) demonstrated the long-term effectiveness of incorporating a social skills module into a 2-week intensive therapy programme for adolescents who stutter, which has now evolved into our communication skills approach.

Rustin and Kuhr (1989) discuss the behaviours which constitute social skills. These include skills such as observation, listening, speaking, meshing, expression of attitudes, social routines, tactics and strategies, non-verbal communication, reinforcement, questioning, reflecting, initiation and closure of contacts, explanations and self-disclosure. Some of these skills are more general than others and most can be broken down into their component parts, for example, single elements, such as looking, nodding, etc.

An additional component, particularly relevant in the area of stuttering, is described by Argyle (1982) as 'meta-perception'. This refers to the fact that interacting persons not only judge others but are also concerned with how they are being judged and that this might significantly affect their own behaviour. For example, it is our experience that many clients have misperceptions of other peoples' views and reactions to their stuttering.

Perception of both the environment and of one's own functioning in relation to the environment is important for understanding social skills. Therefore we have to concern ourselves not only with the client's overt behaviour (e.g. rate and duration of eye-contact) but also with the client's internal state (i.e. feelings, attitudes and perceptions). These cognitive aspects of social skills training are therefore considered as being of equal importance to the behavioural elements.

We use skills training exercises (Rustin and Kuhr, 1989) both to assess the level of social competence the client has achieved to date and to identify particular areas where further training could usefully be carried out. The specific areas with which we are concerned are observation, listening, turntaking, reinforcement and problem-solving. The sequence of these exercises is carefully planned to lead into the negotiation section. Role play exercises afford us the opportunity to teach individual skills which may be missing or poorly developed in the individual's repertoire.

There are difficulties in trying to establish developmental norms for particular social behaviours in adolescents. Our approach is therefore focused on specific social situations which cause particular problems for the individual. This problem-oriented approach to skills training captures the client's imagination and, with the use of role play and problem-solving exercises, provides opportunities to practise and explore alternative coping strategies within the therapy setting. These procedures also contribute to changes in locus of control and ability to empathise.

The skills are taught by use of exercises, video recordings, demonstrations and practice. This continues until the adolescent is confident and competent enough to complete homework tasks based on the newly acquired skills. These homework tasks are essential early transfer activities which will not only reveal difficulties that can be resolved in the clinic but when successfully completed will encourage the client to continue towards the next step.

Observation

Many adolescents who stutter have difficulty maintaining eye-contact and their poor observational skills often lead them to make incorrect judgements about the people with whom they communicate. Directing attention away from the stuttering towards other features of communication and observing the non-verbal behaviour of others alters the nature of the interaction in a positive way.

Listening

Adolescents who stutter are often so preoccupied with their anxiety about speaking that they fail to listen adequately. Instead, they begin to anticipate the difficulty they may have in responding and, as a result, their responses are not only stuttered but also often inappropriate. Chris, aged 15, was asked whether he considered himself to be a 'leader' or 'follower'? His response was 'Yes'. When questioned further, he had understood the question but had not listened to the fact that the question gave a choice.

Focusing attention on what the other person is saying and teaching good listening skills, such as acknowledging, reflecting back, self-disclosure, etc., not only reduces some of the anxiety but also improves the quality of their interaction.

Turntaking

Turntaking is an important feature in initiating, maintaining and ending conversations. It is our experience that many clients who stutter demonstrate some difficulty with this aspect of communication, possibly because their attention is focused on the anticipation of stuttering. The problem is often compounded by poor observation and listening skills. Exercises to improve turntaking skills help the adolescent to become less preoccupied with his stuttering and to concentrate on the conversation in hand.

Praise and reinforcement

As discussed in chapters 1 and 2, teenagers often lack confidence and, for an adolescent who stutters, this will contribute to the problem. Self-confidence develops from a sense of self-worth, this is promoted by the acknowledgement of strengths and personal effort. Increasing self-confidence entails learning how to give and receive praise and encouragement in an appropriate manner. It is important to be able to evaluate performance in a positive way, appreciating good qualities rather than being overwhelmed by failures. An example of this is the use of 'positive statements'. A client identifies something that he does well each day, (e.g. make the bed, dress well, being punctual), and practises making a positive self-statement daily to reinforce the action, *'I really made an effort to look my best today'*, etc. This competence enables them to reinforce both themselves and others which leads to increased feelings of self-worth and confidence.

Problem-solving

The aim is to help the clients learn to make decisions for themselves by understanding that there may be alternative ways of dealing with situations. The ability to solve problems will also enhance their interpersonal skills as it involves observation, listening, turntaking and reinforcement. The technique begins by simply asking a client to describe a current situation that is causing them difficulty, such as buying a bus ticket. We next ask them to brainstorm as many alternative solutions to this problem as they can imagine. We encourage them to think through the consequences of these various alternatives and finally select from the alternatives the one which offers the maximum chance of success. The chosen strategy then can be 'tested out' in reality to see how comfortable it feels and how successful it is in practice. The level of success of the chosen strategy is less important than the elaboration of the client's construing of the possible alternatives.

Negotiation

Negotiation is a higher level skill than problem-solving. It involves having empathy for the other person's point of view, the facility to generate the alternative choices available and an ability to present a reasoned argument on the basis of this understanding. Discussion takes place concerning the continuum of:

Passivity . . . assertion . . . aggression

and how these personality attributes relate to the notion of negotiation.

Being able to negotiate successfully is of particular importance to those who stutter as it helps them to deal more successfully with peer relationships, parents and authority figures.

Good negotiators are less confrontational and more able to assert themselves. This enhances their ability to communicate with others and find mutually agreeable solutions to issues.

Environmental factors

The adolescent who stutters lives within a family and is a member of a social system within which he learns to adapt, therefore therapy can only be truly effective if all aspects of the problem are taken into account. The involvement of the parents as partners in the 'enterprise' provides an ongoing system which can reinforce the effects of the programme while it is in operation and help sustain them following therapy.

It is our belief that parental involvement is an essential prerequisite in the effective management of stuttering in childhood and adolescence. The benefits of involving parents in therapy include: the maintenance of specific skills taught to the child, a greater parental awareness and understanding of the client's problem, and the difficulties which are encountered before, during and after therapy.

The degree and nature of parental involvement does, to some extent, depend on the level of independence that the adolescent has achieved. Our approach with the under 15-year-olds is to have maximum parental involvement in the therapy process (Rustin, 1987). However, in the transitional phase of adolescence a degree of flexibility is required. Commonly, during our intensive group therapy course, a workshop is arranged for all parents where we can explore the nature and development of stuttering, the parents' expectations of therapy and their own philosophies concerning the problem. We also endeavour to put the 'speech' aspect of stuttering into the broader context of general communication skills. During the workshop, the parents observe a number of exercises being carried out by the group members and subsequently are encouraged to attempt for themselves some speech modification strategies, relaxation and social skills exercises. Problem-solving and negotiation techniques are also discussed and a joint exercise is arranged with both groups.

An individual family session is arranged where parents and siblings are invited to discuss and negotiate with the client and therapist a possible role that each might play in contributing to the transfer and maintenance phases of the programme. For example, David, aged 16, in a family session with both parents and his older brother, agreed that his mother could remind him to 'slow down' on a maximum of three occasions per day, five times per week. His father then agreed to remind him to 'take his time', for a maximum of two occasions per day but only four times per week. David did not wish his brother to comment or correct, but asked him to be available once a week to have a conversational practice session. The aim for David was to continue to develop an internal locus of control by reducing the amount of responsibility his family was taking for his stuttering.

In addition to the family session, it is clear that on a day to day basis, involvement with friends and school are increasingly dominant in the adolescent lifestyle. These aspects of life are often the main focus of the stuttering—they are also the most difficult features to address during therapy. Clients may not wish therapists to enter the school environment but frequently wish that the teaching staff had greater understanding of their problem and more productive management strategies. Again, practical examples are given in the next chapter as to how to empower the client through problem-solving, assertiveness and negotiation to tackle these issues for themselves. Where possible, direct contact would be made with the school and additional advice offered to the teaching staff.

The client is also invited to gain peer support by including one close friend in an aspect of therapy. This area is potentially highly productive and is being developed as an integral part of our approach.

These components are discussed in more detail in the following chapter outlining our group intensive programme.

Chapter 5
Intensive Group Management of Adolescents Who Stutter

There follows within this chapter an outline of the intensive 2-week programme which has developed and evolved over a number of years through our own experiences as therapists and through the valuable insights gained from the many young adults who have participated in it.

As we have stressed throughout this book, our approach encompasses a broader range of communication skills than simply fluency. The research carried out by Rustin (1984) indicates that intensive therapy focusing on improvement of overt fluency alone has limited carryover and the gains made in fluency skills are difficult to maintain. This research showed that the more effective and longlasting strategies should include the teaching and practice of a wide range of social communication skills, of which speech modification was a small but important part. We have taken the findings of this research along with those of others in the field of social skills and developed a social skills hierarchy which we have found helpful in the management of the adolescent who stutters.

This hierarchy starts with the basic skills and moves towards increasingly complex, sophisticated skills as follows:

- Observation.
- Listening.
- Turntaking.
- Praise and reinforcement.
- Problem-solving.
- Assertiveness.
- Negotiation.

Other social skills, such as awareness of appropriate proximity, body language, and other non-verbal skills are also discussed and practised where indicated.

Running an intensive fluency course over a 2-week period is a demanding, challenging task which requires clinicians to be highly organised, yet flexible and prepared for all eventualities. Although this can be a daunting prospect for the most experienced therapist, it is, however, a rewarding and invigorating experience as the young adult takes charge of his fluency.

Intensive course procedure

The course aims to:

- Focus on communication skills.
- Gain an insight into the nature of stammering and how to control it.
- Take responsibility for change.
- Experiment with change and consider outcomes.
- Widen experience of effective communication.
- Learn self-reinforcement.
- Increase confidence.

Criteria for acceptance on the course

Certain criteria are essential for the effectiveness of the course:

- Attendance: clients must attend for the duration of the course. We recommend a minimum of 4 hours therapy per day, usually 10 am – 3 pm with a 1-hour lunch break. This age group can cope with extra input, but generally the daily homework tasks add to the amount of time the client is actively involved in the course.
- Parental attendance: one full day is agreed for both parents to attend.
- Language Skills: a good, basic knowledge of English is necessary for the client to benefit from and function in a group setting of this type.
- Follow-up: an intensive course seeks to lay the foundations for improved communication skills. It should be clearly stated when planning the course that follow up sessions are equally important for a continuation of progress. We find that many clients, by the end of the course, are overconfident about their new skills. The follow up sessions will be essential to re-establish new patterns and help clients identify those factors which can make change so difficult to maintain.
- Attitude and motivation: the full assessment and interview procedure is invaluable for ascertaining that all clients accepted on the course have taken full responsibility for the decision to attend.
- Age: this intensive course is most suited to clients within the 15–18 age group.

Organisation of the course

Group size

To some extent this will depend on the accommodation available, however, we have found the optimum number to be eight.

Accommodation

A good sized group room is essential. In addition, a separate staff room and interview room are necessary for individual work, the parents group and family sessions.

Staffing

Three speech and language therapists are required to run a group of six to eight participants in order to conduct individual sessions and assessments. Additional support from speech and language therapy students is recommended. The intensive course provides a valuable teaching environment. Prior training sessions for therapists and students will contribute to the smooth running of the course.

Timing

Although the actual client contact time is usually 4 hours per day, time should be allocated for preparation at the beginning of the day as well as for feedback and discussion at the end of the day. Careful preparation is an essential prerequisite for efficiency and an atmosphere of competence.

Equipment

The following basic equipment is required:

- Work books (Appendix IX).
- Assessment materials.
- Homework sheets (Appendix IX).
- Videotape recorder and monitor.
- Video camera and tapes.
- Audiotape recorder and cassettes.
- Stopwatches and tally counters.
- Calculators.
- Pencils, pens, paper.
- Reading materials.

- Prepared videos of normal dysfluency and communication skills.
- Flip charts, paper and pens.
- Whiteboard or blackboard.
- Reference book for exercises and activities, e.g. Rustin and Kuhr (1989); Rustin (1987); Johnson and Johnson (1975).

Course assessments

Fluency measurement

Assessment of fluency is carried out on the first and last day of the course and at intervals following the course. This measure would include 2 minutes each of reading, monologue and conversation. The conversation section is usually videotape-recorded for additional information concerning social skills.

Changes in fluency can be identified in quantity of dysfluencies, but perhaps more importantly for this age group, the types of dysfluent behaviours are also analysed. We have stressed that total fluency control is not an aim, however, improvement in communication skills and insight into stuttering will increase levels of confidence which, commonly, is reflected by changes in the overall stuttering behaviour (Rustin and Purser, 1983).

Locus of control questionnaire

This gives a baseline score for the client's current status on a measure of internality/externality of his locus of control (Craig, Franklin and Andrews, 1984).

Personal Questionnaire Rapid Scaling Technique

The PQRST (Mulhall, 1977) assessment offers a standardised measure of the client's attitudes towards a variety of personal speaking situations with which they are having difficulty. Apart from offering a test/retest opportunity for monitoring change in attitude and behaviour, this questionnaire is used in the second week of the course to identify those speaking situations which need to be explored, reconstrued and practised by incorporating them into the individual's programme where possible.

Modified Erikson Scale, S-24 Scale

As described in Chapter 2, this seeks to obtain information regarding the client's perceptions of and attitudes towards his dysfluency in terms of 24 different communicative situations.

Character sketches

Kelly (1955) suggested that if you want to know something about someone, you should ask them. He devised an exercise called the 'self characterisation procedure'. This involves inviting the person to write down what he believes to be meaningful about himself. Kelly's instructions were carefully worded as follows:

> I want you to write a character sketch of (name of person, e.g. Harry/ Alice) just as if s/he were the principle character in a play. Write it as it might be written by a friend who knows him or her very intimately and very sympathetically, perhaps better than anyone really could know him or her. Be sure to write it in the third person; for example, start by saying 'Harry/Alice is ...'

These character sketches contribute to the therapists' understanding of the client's view of self and his or her personal world, and can often reveal other aspects concerning the client which have not been previously divulged. They are always helpful in our overall understanding of the client's attitudes about their own strengths and weaknesses. See Appendix X for examples of adolescent self-characterisations.

Social communication checklists

The client is given the opportunity here to evaluate his own social skills. This checklist will be used at intervals throughout the course to monitor progress in areas which may be identified (either by the client or by the therapist) as needing some change (Appendix VI).

Expectations

This is not a formal assessment but an essential step at the beginning of any course. Here the client is required to formalise his thoughts about the prospective course and identify his aspirations, hopes and fears. This is done as an individual paper and pen exercise in the first instance, but is also used as a group activity. It is important to discover the level and nature of expectations in order to clarify what is realistically achievable within the structure of the course. Clearly, if a member of the group has expectations of life changes and total fluency there is likely to be extreme disappointment if these issues are not identified and discussed.

Principles of group management

Group gelling

An effective group depends on the solidarity of its members. Therefore it is essential that the individuals are helped to function as a whole. The foundations for mutual support need to be forged by establishing the common bonds between the group members. The core of group therapy is in the trust and respect that is required from members in order to share their feelings and offer their opinions.

Group gelling is achieved by a combination of structured activities, large and small group discussions, and clear leadership which facilitates ownership of issues under discussion by the group itself.

During sessions the group should be seated in a circle. The seats, where possible, should be of the same size and comfortable. Therapists, students and visitors should be interspersed within the group to avoid the formation of cliques.

It is an important feature of group cohesion that the circle should be reconvened following each activity, that no empty chairs are 'left in' by mistake, and that no group member is allowed to 'sit outside' the circle. The lead therapist should be able to see and hear all group members equally comfortably and vice versa.

As the course progresses, more sophisticated skills are introduced and the demands made upon participants increase. The group will need to be strongly unified and able to support each other. If this element is overlooked as being an essential part of the group dynamic, it will become evident when the demands made upon group members begin to stretch their capabilities and it is likely that individuals, and hence the group, will fail.

Visitors should be introduced and their role explained.

Leadership

The aim is to establish an atmosphere of shared responsibility between the therapists and the group members. Topics which are discussed in small groups will be shared with the large group, the therapist acting as a facilitator to empower the group's natural creativity to generate alternative possibilities to situations. Individuals can then select those ideas which are appropriate to their own circumstances. The group therefore becomes dynamic in solving its own problems.

Homework tasks

Homework is an important part of the structure of the day. These tasks are designed to begin the transference of the skills being established on the course to the clients' real world. Homework tasks are set at the end of each day and written on the homework sheets at the back of the work-book (Appendix IX). The first task for every client each morning is to report back on the completed homework. It is then discussed and forms the basis for the day's activities. Homework that is not done, or partially done, is set for completion during the lunch break and the therapist will invite one of the group members to help the individual complete the task. The therapist will require the individual to report back at the start of the afternoon session.

Insight

The participants should have a clear understanding of the rationale behind the exercises and be given sufficient time to discuss the issues involved and their attitudes towards them. It is helpful to write the outcomes of exercises (e.g. brainstorms) on flipchart paper. These can then be referred to periodically to demonstrate the building blocks of the course.

We have found it useful to display these charts on the wall for easy reference.

Commitment to the group

Occasionally it can happen that a group member is not entirely committed. This may be shown by late arrival, failing to do homework tasks or other behaviours. This will quickly disturb the group solidarity and should be dealt with immediately. There are two possible management strategies:

1. Addressing the problem to the group, who will decide how it should be managed.
2. Giving the individual the opportunity to discuss it with the therapist separately to find a suitable solution.

Workbooks

The workbook is for the client's own use and serves as a concrete record for the contents of the course as a whole and the client's personal observations and assimilations. It is useful for a therapist to check these workbooks periodically to determine progress and ascertain that each client is gathering information appropriately for future reference and has understood the purpose of the work books (Appendix IX).

Structure of the course

The programme is structured around the notion of a daily schedule which incorporates a variety of elements directed towards the overall aims contained within our communication skills approach. The course contains a mixture of didactic presentations, group discussions, group activities, experiential learning and role play.

On a daily basis, the group is given the day plan and a description of the topics which will be covered. These are discussed as part of the total approach.

In its initial phase, the aim is to establish a clearer understanding of the complex nature of communication skills, placing fluency into a holistic context. Participants are given the opportunity to reflect upon and practise such skills, and in this sense, the course has a distinct cognitive–behavioural focus. A range of activities is contained within the programme, these are intended to facilitate the initial development of discrete communication skills, which will gradually become integrated features of our holistic approach. It is not possible to give detailed descriptions of all activities, but all activities which are mentioned in the programme are contained in *Social Skills and the Speech Impaired* (Rustin and Kuhr, 1989), the manual of *The Assessment and Treatment of the Dysfluent Child* (Rustin, 1987) or in *Joining Together: Group Theory and Group Skills* (Johnson and Johnson, 1975).

The following will serve as a framework for the intensive programme we have called the 'Communication Skills Approach'. It is not intended as a rigid regime, rather as a guide to the incremental acquisition of skills for participants. We recognise that each group has its own identity and issues will need to be worked through. The day plans provided in this chapter are intended as a guide only (fig 5.1 etc) and do not need to be rigidly adhered to. We encourage clinicians, therefore, to adapt the programme where appropriate to their own client's needs.

Day 1

Adolescents may feel anxious or insecure within a large, unfamiliar group setting, hence it is important to establish a sense of tolerance and understanding within the group, especially for stuttering behaviour. The focus for this first day will be to gell the group together.

Introductions

A lead therapist should be identified for the first part of the morning, who will take responsibility for the welcome and for the introduction of the participants including the clients and all others involved. Each person should have a clearly written name badge.

Facts about the course

The first session aims to provide factual information in order for the group to become acquainted with the surroundings and the basic rules that need to be established. This includes an orientation to the host building, explicit reference to the times of the group, punctuality, lunchtimes, facilities, etc. A broad overview of the course is given which sets the scene for the following two weeks. An overview of the first day is

DAY ONE

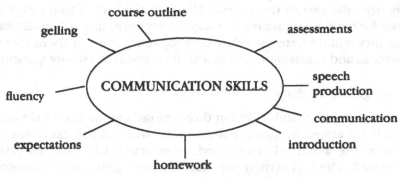

Times
AM

10.00 Introductions- Therapists
Students
Clients
(Making sure each has a name badge)
Introductions to the Course
i) Times of the Group - Importance of Punctuality
ii) Orientation to the Building - Lunch Areas, Toilets etc.
iii) Overview of the Course:
– Looking at Communication Skills
– Fluency - Understanding stuttering better
– Importance of open dialogue and discussion
– Remember- its OK to stutter here
– Practical exercises and opportunities for real experience of communication in a wide range of contexts
– Parental Involvement
– Workbooks
– Visitors to the Course
iv) Overview of the First Day
– Assessments in order to establish a baseline and measure progress
– Initial written work, including Self Rating Scales

10.15 GROUP GELLING ACTIVITY:
i) The Name Game - with a caller
ii) Find out Three Things

10.30 WRITTEN WORK AND INDIVIDUAL FLUENCY ASSESSMENTS
– What are your expectations of the Course?
– PQRST
– Social Communication Skills Rating Scale
– Self Characterisations
–Locus of Control Questionaire

11.30 Feedback expectations of Course onto Flipchart and discussion

11.50 GROUP GELLING ACTIVITY
– Name Game

12.00 LUNCH

THINGS TO REMEMBER
– Make explicit statement about fact that it is OK to Stutter
– Make sure all have made good progress on written exercises

PM

1.00 WARM UP ACTIVITY
Fruit Salad

1.10 BRAINSTORM:
" *COMMUNICATION* "

1.30 SPEECH PRODUCTION - How Speech is Made: X-ray Video and Sectional anatomical model of head and larynx

1.50 BRAINSTORM:
What can go wrong with Speech? "

2.10 Written Individual Work with therapist/student
i) " What happens when I stutter? "
ii) " What can I do about it? "

2.30 Feedback to larger group - Discuss similarities and differences

2.45 GROUP ACTIVITY
The Introduction Game:– 'I'm.......and this is......'

2.55 BRAINSTORM
" What is Fluency? "
(Video of normally dysfluent speaker)

3.15 HOMEWORK:
Observe two people at home - Rate their fluency on a scale of I-10
What makes them fluent/not fluent?

3.20 Good news/bad news

THINGS TO REMEMBER
– Make sure brainstorms are written in workbooks and recorded on central file -
– Make sure expectations are entered into personal workbooks

Figure 5.1 The communication skills approach: day 1.

also helpful. Here, emphasis is given to the fact that it is a fairly atypical day from the rest of the course. The lead therapist should explain the need for baseline measures in a way the young adults will understand so that they will tolerate the relatively long time which is spent on written exercises and assessments. Opportunity is given to ask any questions.

Group gelling activity

'The Name Game' and 'Find out three things' are the first of the activities which are aimed at group cohesion. As with all the exercises on the course, the activity is explained, conducted and then its rationale discussed. The first activity will start the gelling process and encourage the recognition and memorising of group members' names. We have found it beneficial to have a 'caller' for the names at this stage, i.e. a therapist who calls out the names rather than expecting the clients out to call their own names. This ensures that the demands of the activity do not outstrip the capacities of the youngsters at this stage of the programme and that no-one is left out. The second activity ensures that course participants begin to interact with each other and will help to establish some similarities and commonalities for the formation of early networks.

Written exercises and assessments

These are described on pp. 74 and 75 and are baseline measures. Some of them will be for use during the course, others will be readministered at the end of the course or in the follow up sessions to monitor progress and identify changes. The written exercise concerning expectations of the course will be the first opportunity for open discussion within the group. Some clients have quite unrealistic aims and it is important that the whole group works towards creating a realistic consensus in order to avoid disappointment. Following the discussion, each group member should reconsider their original list and write their expectations in the appropriate section in their workbooks.

Group gelling activity

'The Name Game' is repeated before lunch.

Lunch

At the first lunch break, the therapist will confirm that all participants know where to go, etc. We recommend that the group goes in twos or threes and that no-one is left on their own for the hour.

Group gelling/warm-up activity

Self-explanatory.

Brainstorm

'Communication'. This brainstorm technique (Priestly et al., 1978) is used frequently throughout the course. It is explained to the group that the aim is to generate as many ideas as possible on a given topic. The rules are as follows:

* Aim for quantity not quality.
* Do not judge the ideas as their value can be assessed later.
* Let the mind wander – wild and quirky ideas can turn out to be winners.
* Build on the ideas of others, expanding and adding to ideas already offered.

The topic should be written at the top of the blackboard or large sheet of paper and all the ideas listed underneath. Afterwards the ideas are grouped or numbered in order of perceived importance. The purpose of this exercise is to develop a more holistic view of the skills required for good communication and to start to shift the focus away from fluency by placing it in the context of a broader range of communication skills.

The lead therapist should aim to elicit the key elements of the 'communication skills' hierarchy: Observation (eye-contact, looking); Listening (paying attention, understanding, reflecting); Turntaking (pausing); Reinforcement (praising), as well as Speech skills. (See Appendix XI for an example of a recent groups' brainstorm.) This provides the foundations for future work on the course and can be used as an important reference point throughout the programme. A further consideration for the lead therapist in the early stages of this course is to ensure that every member of the group contributes. To fulfil this aim, the lead therapist will ask each client in turn for a suggestion before the brainstorm becomes a 'free for all'.

Speech production

This takes the form of a presentation and provides a useful framework to enable clients to understand the mechanics of speech production, the breakdown in terms of stuttering in general and their own particular pattern of dysfluency.

Brainstorm

'What can go wrong with speech?' This enables clients to reflect fully upon the wide range of communication difficulties to be found in the general population and helps them to appreciate a little more about the nature of their own communication difficulties. (Appendix XI, for example.)

Written exercise

- 'What happens when I stutter?'
- 'What can I do about it?

Clients work individually with a therapist to identify the specifics of their own stuttering behaviour, as well as any strategies or techniques which they may currently use in order to control it. This is then shared with the group which not only serves to get stuttering 'out into the open' but also to enhance and develop a clearer sense of group identity as many problems are shared and similar experiences identified by course participants, which serves to consolidate the group further.

Group activity

For example, 'The Introduction Game'. This is another opportunity to develop networks within the group. Participants should be directed to pair up with somebody with whom they have not already worked.

Brainstorm

'What is fluency?' This is a powerful brainstorm as it serves to tune participants into looking at fluency in a broader sense and is another step towards facilitating a clearer understanding of their own stuttering behaviour. The therapist will aim to elicit those factors which will be introduced for the 'fluency' aspect of communication skills, e.g. rate, flow and easy onsets. It is also important to discover the client's inaccurate perception concerning fluency (e.g. no mistakes, no repetitions, no blocks, always able to say the word you want, total control, etc.). At this stage it is valuable to show a video of a normally fluent person which demonstrates the common disfluencies of speech. This is often a real 'eye-opener'!

Debriefing and homework

The afternoon is completed by regrouping the clients as usual into the circle and providing a brief summary of the day, inviting comments and any questions they may have at this stage. Homework tasks are set and, as with any homework activity, it is essential that the clients write this down so that they have a clear and accurate understanding of what is required.

Day 2

Day 2 (see Fig 5.2) focuses upon identifying fluency factors and introduces the first element of social skills ,'observation'.

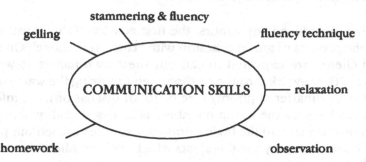

DAY TWO

stammering & fluency

gelling

fluency technique

COMMUNICATION SKILLS — relaxation

homework   observation

AM

10.00 GROUP ACTIVITY
    – *Name Game - all calling*
10.10 Homework Feedback
10. 30 Introduction to Fluency Factors:
    i) Re-introduce Brainstorm from yesterday -
    ~What is Fluency?~
    ii) Introduce Fluency Technique
    Slowing
    Flowing
    Easy Onset
    iii) Therapist demonstrates each of the
    above factors in isolation and in combina-
    tion
    iv) When indicated introduce
    Breathing
    Soft Contacts
    Intonation
10.45 Individual or paired technique work with
    therapist/student
    – enter initial individual fluency factors in
    workbooks
11.00 Introduce Social Skills:
    – Reintroduce Brainstorm - " Communica-
    tion " from yesterday
    – Focus on OBSERVATION

GROUP ACTIVITY:
    " Change Three Things "

GROUP DISCUSSION:
    " Importance of Observation " - write up
    onto flip chart paper
    (Discuss how yesterday's homework was
    involved in this aspect of communication)

11.30 ROLE PLAY - by Therapists:
    Poor Social Communication Skills
    – Poor eye contact/observation
    – Not listening
    – Interrupting/asking too many questions
    – Monotonous voice

    – Disagreeing negation
11.50 GROUP ACTIVITY:
    " Eye Contact Game "
    (Page 126, Social Skills and the Speech
    Impaired)
12.00 LUNCH

THINGS TO REMEMBER
    – Put up previous day's and today's Brain-
    storms on wall
    – Make sure that the Brainstorms are writ-
    ten up in workbooks by end of the day
PM
1.00 GROUP GAME
    " *Eye Swap Chairs* "
1.10 Technique practice- Individually/pairs with
    therapist revise fluency factors where appro-
    priate
1.25 RELAXATION
    –*Body Maps: Identifying points of tension*
1.45 OBSERVATION GAME
    – *'Pass the Pens '*
2.00 RELAXATION EXERCISE
2.15 Fluency Factors practice
2.30 OBSERVATION GAME
    –" *Changing Statues* "
2.45 GOOD NEWS / BAD NEWS
    HOMEWORK:
    " Who is a good communicator at home?
    Why?"
    Observe a tense/relaxed person

FLUENCY PRACTICE

THINGS TO REMEMBER
    –Keep focussing back to observation skills
    - Always check out that clients have under-
    stood purpose of exercise

Figure 5.2 The communication skills approach: day 2

Activity and homework feedback

Having introduced any visitors, the first activity of the morning contin-ues the process of group cohesion with 'The Name Game'. On this occa-sion clients are expected to call out their own names as well as the others'. Homework is routinely discussed following the warm-up/gelling activity as a matter of priority (see p. 76 for discussion), the information brought back by the group members is analysed and, where possible, reference is made to the brainstorms or exercises carried out previously and issues noted by the therapists which will be salient for the current day's discussions.

Introduction to fluency factors: slowing, flowing and easy onsets

The brainstorm from the previous day is reintroduced – '**What is fluency?**' and these aspects identified from the flipchart. A therapist demonstrates each of these factors, first in isolation, then in single words and finally in phrases and sentences to illustrate the fluency factors in practice. Emphasis is placed on making the fluency factors sound as natural as possible. For a small number of clients, a further three factors may be introduced later: breathing, soft contacts and normal intonation. It is recommended that in the early stages the first three elements should be the starting point for experimenting with speech control.

Individual session

Experimentation and identification of personal fluency factors. This session allows each client to work individually with a therapist to select the right combination of fluency factors which modify his stuttering behaviours and offer strategies for control. At this stage it is helpful to have an experienced therapist available to monitor each client's under-standing and use of personal fluency factors. This also affords the oppor-tunity to help clients distinguish between this approach and other speech modification techniques which they may have been instructed in previously but which may have been unsuccessful for a variety of reasons (see p. 60 for discussion). This phase is experimental and one following which the client should have a clearer notion of those individual fluency factors upon which he needs to concentrate in order to achieve an acceptable sense of personal control. The client enters his fluency factors in the workbook as a reminder (Appendix IX).

Introduction to social skills

The brainstorm concerning communication is reintroduced at this junc-ture. The lead therapist will facilitate a discussion concerning the importance of observation skills. This provides an entrée into the next group activity 'The Observation Game – Change Three Things'. On completion, each person is invited to tell the group how he got on with the task and to explain any difficulties that may have arisen. Each person is also asked which role they preferred in the pair. A group discussion then follows where the purpose of the exercise is analysed and the therapist checks that each person has understood. Key points from this discussion should be clearly displayed as a reminder.

Poor communication skills: role play by therapists (or video presentation)

Examples demonstrating inadequate or poor skills in each of the following areas: eye-contact, observation, listening skills, turntaking, and intonation. Each 'mini scenario' shows a shortcoming in one specific area and participants comment upon what they consider might be the weakness after each enactment.

Group activity

'The Eye Contact Game'. This continues to focus on eye-contact and observational skills. This activity is discussed and key points highlighted for future reference.

Lunch

Therapists may wish to check again that the group looks after its members during the lunch break. Unfinished homework tasks are completed during this period as before.

Group activity

'Eye Swap Chairs': group gelling continues and as each activity is completed, reference is made to the purpose and progress.

Individual session

Revision of personal fluency factors with each client. An individual programme of fluency work is now introduced. The first phase will involve the therapist and client practising together through the stages of: therapist 'modelling' the target word, followed by practice in unison and, finally, the client on his own, as shown in the workbook. At this stage the therapist will correct, explain, and demonstrate as required until the client has identified and is able to show that his speech can be controlled with the fewest possible modification strategies. At this stage, too, for the client where slow, flow and easy onsets are insufficient, additional features, including soft contacts, breath control and intonational work, may be introduced. The main programme of fluency work is not introduced until the client has achieved success throughout Phase 1. Fluency practice generally is carried out in frequent, short episodes throughout the first week (for example, 3×15 minutes per session).

Relaxation

(See p. 65.) Body maps help clients to identify the areas where muscular tension is experienced when in difficult speaking situations. A discussion of the 'normality' of a certain amount of tension in a person's life is useful. The 'fight and flight' theory of self-preservation can form part of the discussion. The intention is to demonstrate that tension does not cause the stuttering but excessive amounts may be the result of predicted problems before the stuttering. Each person identifies their own areas of tension and a group discussion can then illustrate the similarities and differences within the group.

Group activity

The focus on observation skills continues with another group activity which requires each participant to concentrate on honing their abilities in this area.

Relaxation exercise

This is the first time that the concept of relaxation is directly introduced and it will now become a feature of the day to day programme. The therapist will discuss relaxation from a physiological standpoint. It is essential in a programme of this type that new elements are introduced through discussion to establish the client's 'ownership' of each aspect. The client who has insight into the purpose of each activity will be a more active participant and therefore more successful in acquiring new skills. It is important to point out that relaxation is a new skill which takes time to acquire; that some will find it easier than others; some will find it more beneficial than others, but with practice, all will find a practical advantage.

Individual fluency practice

A continuation of individual sessions from the workbook.

Observation game

This aspect of communication skills has now been thoroughly examined and participants will be actively construing their own abilities in this area.

Good news/bad news

A structured round-up of the day is provided within this exercise. Each client is asked to report on what the 'Good news' has been for them during the day (aspects which they found beneficial, interesting, etc) and anything that was 'Bad news' (activities which have not been useful, poor progress on particular aspects, etc).

Homework

Here we pose the question *'Who is a good communicator at home?'* *'Why?'* As well as this they are asked to observe a tense or relaxed person and to give reasons why they have made that judgement. The purpose of these exercises is to focus the client's own observation skills in order that they can become more objective concerning the communicative behaviour of others and the variation between individuals.

Day 3

The focus of the third day continues to enhance the fluency skills through the individual programmes, to build upon the observation skills practised yesterday and to introduce the next element of listening in the communication skills approach (see Fig. 5.3).

Homework feedback

At this stage the group skills will be developing and the homework feedback time is an opportunity for the group to begin to develop independent interactive skills which are not therapist-led. Participants are invited to form small groups and to nominate a spokesperson to feedback to the main group on behalf of their subgroup. The foundation skills of assertiveness and negotiation are thus being introduced at an entirely practical level. This process is then openly discussed in the main group after the homework has been reviewed.

Brainstorm

The group is reintroduced to the brainstorm of communication skills and the topic of listening is drawn out. The brainstorm specifically on the topic of listening is written up and discussed. The ideas are intended to help everyone broaden their perspective on this skill.

Group activity

'The Listening Game'. The purpose of this game is to demonstrate how difficult it is to listen accurately. It also provides an opportunity to teach

DAY THREE

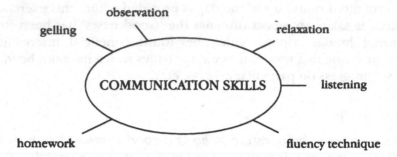

AM

10.00 GROUP ACTIVITY
10.10 Homework Feedback

10.30 GROUP ACTIVITY:
       –THE LISTENING GAME
       (Observer/Speaker/Listener)
11.00 Feedback on Purpose of Activity: Group
       Discussion
       " Why is Listening Important for Good
       Communication ? "
11.20 Relaxation Exercise
11.35 Fluency Practice

11.50 GROUP ACTIVITY:
       " Who started the Cesture?"

12.00 LUNCH

FLUENCY PRACTICE

THINGS TO REMEMBER
       – Make sure all Brainstorms are written up
       in workbooks
       – Individual fluency factors in workbooks
       have been written down in workbooks

1.00   GROUP ACTIVITY:
       " Who started the gesture? "
       –Observation/listening

1.10   CIRCLE OF CONFIDENCE
       and
       GROUP DISCUSSION:
       How do you know whether someone is
       listening?
1.35   Relaxation and Fluency Factors

1.55   GROUP ACTIVITY:
       " Breaking into the Circle "
2.10   Feedback and discussion about this exercise

2.20   GROUP ACTIVITY:
       " Sculpting" - Proximity/ personal space
       - Resolution of problem
       relationship/situations

2.40   GROUP DISCUSSION:
       What was the purpose of above exercise?

2.50   Good News / Bad News
       Homework:
       Who does the most interrupting at home?
       " "   " "   listening   " "
       " "   " "   talking   " "

FLUENCY PRACTICE

THINGS TO REMEMBER

Figure 5.3 The communication skills approach: day 3

clients how to be critical and to evaluate an exercise fairly, as well as how to give or receive criticism and praise appropriately. A full discussion is important for the appreciation of the significance of acquiring good listening skills. The therapist will elicit from the group members that quality of listening is more important than quantity. An elaboration of each member's perception of how they felt in each role in the exercise is valuable. The observer in the triad may report difficulties in listening because of the positioning and consequent lack of eye-contact, and a feeling of perhaps being excluded, although often the role is also perceived as easier because one is not the main focus of attention. This can be picked up and related to stuttering. The listener may have misinterpreted some aspects of the story, which can be irritating and frustrating to the storyteller and would be worthy of discussion related to real life experiences.

Relaxation

Further experience is now offered to build the client's repertoire of understanding those aspects over which he can start to gain some control.

Individual fluency session

By this stage, it would be anticipated that Phase 1 will have been completed and the clients will have progressed on to the programme steps themselves. At this stage it is important that the therapists withdraw their advice and guidance. This can be extremely difficult for a therapist to do, essentially therapists are 'helpers' by nature. The objective now is that the client takes responsibility for his own fluency. In an attempt to focus this in as defined a manner as possible, a behavioural approach is selected. The programme steps are designed to increase the length and complexity of the task in small steps. The client is stopped for fluency breaks and the step repeated until successful. When the fluency begins to break down, the client will only progress when he remembers the fluency factors. Our concern here is that if the therapist reinstructs the client in the fluency factors then she is taking over the responsibility from the client. *Progress is killed by kindness!* The modes of reading, monologue and conversation are worked through systematically until the client has achieved the final step of 2 minutes in each mode.

Group activity

This will be selected to continue to build on observation and listening skills.

Lunch break

Homework tasks which had not been completed will be re-instructed now.

Group activity
Group discussion

'Circle of Confidence/Cycle of Stuttering'. This involves a presentation to elaborate the growing understanding of our broader communication skills approach. The aim is to address the vicious circle which is involved with the maintenance of stuttering behaviours in contrast to the 'Circle of Confidence' whereby increasingly effective communication skills will take the focus away from the stuttering itself moving towards the more productive notions of self-esteem. The overall objective is to remind the participants that we are not aiming for a cure but seeking an effective way of managing the problem (Appendix XIII).

Review of listening

'How do you know whether someone is listening?' This topic can be usefully discussed in small groups first then fed back to the main group by a spokesperson. This activity has four purposes:

- Broadening the client's perspective.
- Practising independent discussions.
- Giving each client the opportunity to lead groups.
- Turntaking.

Relaxation

The physiological method (p. 65) is adaptable to being taught in a variety of physical positions, e.g. lying down, sitting, standing, walking. As the programme continues, it is useful to change the positions in order to demonstrate that 'quick' relaxation can be achieved in different settings. Transferring the relaxation skills within the group now becomes practicable and therapists can draw clients' attention to tense postures, or physical signs of anxiety. The relaxation sessions are scheduled before the fluency control practice to emphasise this point.

Individual fluency session

The individual programme steps are continued.

Brainstorm

'Why is turntaking important in communication?' This will focus on some ideas that have already been mentioned and will identify some of the particular difficulties facing the person who stutter. We have already demonstrated, by example to the group, that participation by every member on this course is necessary. At this point we need to highlight the reasons why turntaking is seen as a significant element.

Group activity

'**Breaking into the circle.**' This is not seen as a game but rather an exercise which clearly demonstrates the emotional aspects of being unable to break into a group and the efforts to which one might have to go in order to succeed. The feelings experienced within this activity by the person excluded, correlate with the experiences of the person who stutters. The discussion which follows expands the notion of the importance of turntaking and of being included. This topic will be developed over the next few days.

Group activity

'**Sculpting**'. This activity will begin to focus the clients towards the precursors of problem-solving: at this stage it will also demonstrate aspects of non-verbal skills, such as proximity, posture, and group dynamics.

Group discussion

Follows the 'sculpting' exercise and analyses its purpose and the outcome.

Good news/bad news

This is now a feature on a daily basis. Not only does it afford an opportunity for each group member to demonstrate his feelings of progress and concerns about certain aspects, it also presents an ideal chance for the therapists to feedback to the group from their point of view.

Homework

This is an observation task which is intended to enhance each client's objectivity. In addition, clients are asked to specify some personal commitment to fluency practice. It would be suggested that the choice would depend on the stage that he has reached in their programme and can be done on their own at home. The emphasis here would be that the home fluency practice should be carried out using the fluency factors.

Day 4

This fourth day continues the themes of observation, listening, turntaking and now introduces, in a more formal sense, praise and reinforcement, assertion and negotiation.

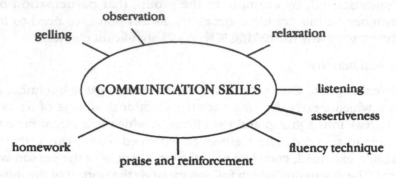

DAY FOUR

AM
10.00 GROUP ACTIVITY:
       – Discuss homework in small groups -
       nominate a spokesperson to feedback to
       main group
10.10 Feedback of Homework - How did you
       nominate the spokesperson?
10.30 Fluency Practice

10.45 GROUP ACTIVITY:
       " Let me in: Triads "
       –Role Play; Turn taking
       Group feedback: Purpose of activity?

11.10 GROUP ACTIVITY:
       " Praise Game"
       Feedback to group: What praise did they
       receive? What was reaction?
       Round up of importance of praise and self
       reinforcement

11.20 GROUP ACTIVITY:

       " Lets go on a picnic - I chose you because "
       Feedback and round up to group

11.45 GROUP FLUENCY ACTIVITY:
       "I went to market and I bought a......"

11.55 LUNCHTIME TASK:
       - Pay a compliment/praise someone and
       note their reaction

FLUENCY PRACTICE

THINGS TO REMEMBER
       Make a video of activity to show parents
       tomorrow

PM
1 00   GROUP DISCUSSION:
       Of lunchtime task and nomination of
       spokesperson

1.10   GROUP ACTIVITY:
       " Finding out "
       - Find out three new things about each
       other.
       Reporting back: take turns to report back
       one thing each upto three

1.35   BRAINSTORM:
       " What is Assertiveness? "
       - discuss Passivity...Assertion...Aggression
       continuum
       - Advantages and disadvantages of passivity
       aggression
       Where are you now? Where would you like
       to be?
2.05   Relaxation/Fluency Practice

2.35   GROUP ACTIVITY:
       " Desert Island "- Assertion and Negotiation
       i) eg 4 groups of 3
       ii) eg I group of 4 representatives
       iii) Feedback on how reps performed

3.05   Good news/bad news
       Homework: Try using fluency factors in
       activity of your choice
       Praise someone at home- note their reaction
3.15   Close

FLUENCY PRACTICE

THINGS TO REMEMBER
       Video desert island activity
       Explain format for parents day for tomorrow
       Carry forward any items not covered today

Figure 5.4 The communication skills approach: day 4

Warm up/gelling

Homework

Participants again form small groups to discuss their homework and nominate a spokesperson to feedback to the main group on their behalf. This again contributes to the more complex aspects of communication skills of assertion and negotiation. The emerging issues are discussed as is the importance of objectivity. The therapist's aim is to elicit information concerning the variation in others' communication skills.

Fluency practice

As participants near the end of the first phase of the programme steps, paired practice can be introduced.

Group activity

Topic: **turntaking 'Let Me In'.** The activity comprises role play in triads. Each is allocated a role: 'mother', 'father' and 'child'. The 'parents' are instructed to conduct a conversation whilst not allowing the child to interrupt them. The task for the 'child' is to do everything possible to break into this conversation and gain their attention. The discussion following this elaborates the importance of turntaking. It is useful to direct the participants' attention to their feelings in each role and the methods they employed to 'keep the child out', or 'to break in'. The therapist will ensure that successful turntaking skills include eye-contact, listening and observing but not necessarily verbal skills on their own. (Note: role play is a powerful tool which can engender considerable emotions. It is important, therefore, to 'de-role' each of the participants following the completed exercise.)

Group activity

Topic: **praise 'The Praise Game'.** The aim is to discover if group members are able to make positive remark to each other and if they can accept them. Participants split into pairs, their task is to hold a conversation for 3 minutes, during which time each participant must pay a compliment to, or make a positive statement about their partner. The main group then reconvenes and each participant is to relate the compliment or praise that they received. Their partner is then to report what reaction was gained from the person receiving the compliment – was it accepted or rejected? The feedback explores the difficulties encountered in making positive statements and in receiving them. Only when all responses have been gained should the lead therapist summarise the importance of giving and receiving praise. A specific issue which needs to be addressed is the sincerity of the praise, which should be relevant and fitting. Specific reference should be made at this point to those pairs who did not appear to carry out the task correctly and they are invited to try out the task again.

Group activity

Topic: **praise and reinforcement,** e.g. 'I would like to go on a picnic with you because ...'

Group fluency activity

'*I went to market and I bought a ...*' At this stage the transfer of the personal fluency factors is initiated through rote group speech practice. A game of this type puts little stress on language skills and is designed to focus on an individual's first attempt to maintain fluency within a group setting.

Lunchtime task

Pay a compliment/praise someone and note their reaction.

Group discussion

Concerning the lunchtime task.

Group activity

Topic: **listening, eye-contact, observation, turntaking, assertion,** 'Find Out Three New Things'. Discussion about the different skills that are involved in conversational moves as above.

Group discussion

Topic: **'Assertiveness'.** This significant theme will be considered in some detail. It is vital to clarify the difference between assertion and aggression. We propose the use of a continuum:

Passivity . . . Assertion . . . Aggression

A brainstorm can be used for each notion or small group discussions could debate the continuum within the 'Advantages and disadvantages' dimensions. Frequently, our clients have experienced difficulties in this area, tending to react to difficult situations at one or other end of the extremes on the continuum. The lead therapist would ensure that the discussion resulted in assertiveness being the ideal, which is underpinned by the communication skills approach. Each client is invited to consider where he is on the continuum and where he would like to be.

Relaxation

Fluency practice

Group activity

Topic: **assertion and negotiation**, 'Desert Island'. This activity is videotape recorded, and is used to give instant feedback concerning individual member's own ratings of their communication skills. The social skills self rating scale (Appendix VI) can be used at this point to consider those areas in which the young adults feel they do well and those aspects which they feel could be improved upon. The use of a videotape recorder offers an important opportunity for the young adults to learn self-monitoring and self-reinforcement skills. The lead therapist, when reviewing the videotape recording, is concerned to help individuals look for the 'good news' first (i.e. those aspects of their performance which were positive), before identifying aspects for change and development.

Good news/bad news

Homework

Fluency practice and a praise exercise.

Day 5

(Parents' group – simultaneous workshop.) The focus of the day will be the introduction to problem-solving. Effective problem-solving depends on the foundation skills of listening, observation, turntaking, praise and assertiveness. The aim for the parents will be to offer the rationale for the communication skills approach, through experiential activities and discussion. Following a separate introduction to the day for the parents, the groups are brought together to offer the parents a brief opportunity to observe the client group participating in an activity. The groups then work separately until the last half hour of the afternoon.

The parents' observation session requires careful planning. It is explained that whilst the group is involved in an activity, the parents will be invited to seat themselves in the outer circle behind their own children. Their job is to observe only. They will not be invited to participate, comment or otherwise attract attention. It is emphasised that the client group will be very anxious about being scrutinised, and therefore it is incumbent upon the parents to respect these rules.

The objective of the observation session is to broaden the parents' perspective on the function of the group and the similarities and differ-

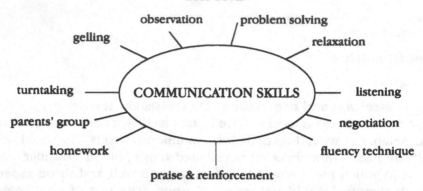

DAY FIVE

observation   problem solving

gelling   relaxation

turntaking ——— COMMUNICATION SKILLS ——— listening

parents' group   negotiation

homework   fluency technique

praise & reinforcement

AM		PM	
10.00	Feedback of Homework: Group Discussion and spokesperson Parents out receiving own introduction to the day	1.00	Feedback from morning as whole group - how was am with parents? outline of what is happening in parents group in pm.
10.15	Parents join main group as observers		Check that lunchtime tasks were completed.

AM

10.00 Feedback of Homework:
Group Discussion and spokesperson
Parents out receiving own introduction to
the day

10.15 Parents join main group as observers

GROUP FLUENCY/TURN TAKING ACTIVITY:
" The Microphone Game "
Can only speak when you have the
micro phone

10.35 GROUP ACTIVITY:
" What is my job?"

11.05 GROUP ACTIVITY:
PROBLEM SOLVING: Therapists problem e.g
Can't get up in the mornings

11.35 GROUP ACTIVITY:
" I'm going to a party and I'm going to
wear.... "
(Rule game: Observation, listening, problem solving and fluency)

11.55 GROUP ACTIVITY:
" Praise Came "

12.05 Lunchtime task with parents
i) One positive statement to each family
member from
each family member
ii) Think of a problem you would like to
solve

PM

1.00 Feedback from morning as whole group -
how was am with parents?
outline of what is happening in parents
group in pm.
Check that lunchtime tasks were completed.

1.30 GROUP ACTIVITY:
" The Moon Base Game " Negotiation,
Assertion,
Problem Solving

2.30 GROUP ACTIVITY:
"Spin the Plate"

2.35 Set Homework: Fluency Practice
Observation Task
Prepare a list of difficult speaking
situations they would like to practice
Choose solutions from problem solve
Report back on Monday

2.45 GROUP ACTIVITY:

PROBLEM SOLVE
Parents rejoin the group - Parents and
Young Adults
commence problem solve in Triads with
therapist attached to each family

FLUENCY PRACTICE

THINGS TO REMEMBER

Figure 5.5 The communication skills approach: day 5

ences between the group members who stutter. Despite the anxiety that the observation session will engender, the benefits for the parents' group far outweigh the disadvantages.

For the adolescent group the normal format of the day is in place.

Homework feedback

Small groups, checking that a new spokesperson is identified each day.

Parents' observation session

Group fluency activity.

Introduction to problem-solving

(See p. 68.) Here it may be advisable to conduct the first 'problem-solve' with a non-speech related topic 'Not being able to get up in the morning'. (Note: a problem-solve must concern a real, identified problem from one of the group members.) The rest of the morning session focuses on activities which involve observation, listening, problem- solving and fluency.

Lunch break

Both groups are instructed in a lunchtime task.

Feedback

1. Discussion about lunch time task.
2. Discussion about parental observation session.

Group activity

Topic: **negotiation, assertion, problem-solving.** This activity is videotape recorded and, again, provides important material for discussion of foundational skills development on an individual basis and for the more advanced skills concerning problem-solving, negotiation and assertiveness.

Homework

For the weekend:
* Fluency practice, set up for each individual according to their progress on the programme.
* To identify a list of speaking situations which are problematic and which they would like to have the opportunity of practising.
* Finish the joint problem-solve (see below) with their parents, identifying the order in which the solutions will be attempted and trying them out if possible.

Group Activity with Parents

Parents re-join the group and conduct a problem-solve within the family group (usually triads). The therapists will monitor this activity.

Parents' group

Following the initial observation session, the parents' group convenes in a separate room with one of the therapists. Labels for names should be worn.

Our experience with parents' groups suggests that a 1-day only workshop limits the number of topics that can be covered. Two days is recommended but often difficult to implement.

In order to attain maximum benefit, it is essential that group cohesion is achieved. Thus a mixture of practical exercises, demonstrations and presentations may be used.

Gelling Game

'Introduction Game'. This game is conducted in exactly the same way as described on Day 1 of the course. As usual, a discussion follows which elicits the rationale for the activity. Parents are invited to share with the group how they felt about speaking out in front of the group for the first time. Initially some will express feelings of nervousness, shyness, anxiety or fear concerning, for example, not being able to do the task well enough in front of strangers. This is followed by a sense of relief as the therapist points out the commonality of these feelings. The exercise serves not only to help the group initiate conversations with each other but also to consider how their own teenager with the additional stuttering problem might feel in the same circumstances.

Expectations of the day/expectations of intensive group

As with all groups, it is important to understand their hopes and fears for the day. This activity is usually carried out in small groups, a leader nominated and ideas subsequently shared with the whole group. The advantage of group discussion is that any unrealistic expectations will be dealt with by either the subgroup or large group. The therapist's skill is in not offering answers but throwing problems back to the group for clarification and debate. Group solutions are far more powerful than dictate. These two discussions on expectations are sequential. The first will elicit information about the knowledge they would like to gain and the problems they may wish to discuss. The second will establish their beliefs about therapy and the nature of stuttering. The debate should aim to re-establish that there is no single answer to the problem of stuttering.

The results form the basis for the following topics.

Nature of stuttering and the nature of adolescence

The first can take the form of a didactic presentation. The facts of stuttering are introduced, which may be revision for most of the parents. A brief presentation of the research on aetiology may be included, but more importantly the development of stuttering should be elaborated. The second topic, adolescence, is ripe for a brainstorming exercise. Parents usually have very many thoughts and ideas to contribute. The therapist's role initially is to identify the various themes concerning, for example, changes in self, pressures and independence. Then she can highlight the number of negative and positive ideas which have been elicited. This can now usefully be compared with the brainstorm from their own adolescents as well as one entitled 'How Parents View Adolescence – The Group's Ideas'. (See Appendices XIV, XV and XVI). It commonly occurs that the parents' and other adults' perception are negatively weighted, whereas the teenagers' themselves may have a very different viewpoint.

Small group exercise

'Your Teenager's Stutter': this further discussion in small groups, offers the opportunity to the parents of discovering the similarities and differences which occur as well as the range. This offers a further occasion for the therapist to identify the complexity and individuality of stuttering. (Note: parents often have a great deal to say on this matter and the therapist may have to curtail the discussion due to time constraints.)

Feedback to flipchart

The similarities and differences are summarised.

Brainstorm

'Communication Skills': the therapist's task here is to make sure that the elements of the communication skills approach are elicited.

Communication skills approach

An overview of the components of this approach is offered. Where possible, ideas which were generated from the previous exercises are pointed out and linked to: the effects that stuttering has on social interaction; the behavioural consequences of the fear of communication; the lack of practice in social relationships and the inevitable paucity of skills in problem-solving and negotiation. A presentation of the results of previous research into the use of social skills training with fluency modification strategies confirms the rationale behind this broad therapeutic approach.

Brainstorm

'What is Fluency?': this is another important brainstorm for the group. The therapist will bear in mind that the chances of the therapy group members achieving normal fluency is reducing. Therefore it is productive for the therapist to highlight the continuum and range of the so-called 'normal fluency'. (Note: as each activity is completed the therapist should point out that each of these exercises has been part of the main therapy programme.)

Speech modification

This practical exercise includes the programme steps of modelling, unison and group only. Concentrating on 'slow', 'flow' and 'easy onsets'. A further paired group exercise to gain experience in trying to maintain a conversation and monitor the speech modification aspects simultaneously is effective. A group discussion can then identify the difficulties the group members experienced in fulfilling the task and therefore better understand the burden that is imposed on their teenager when a fluency technique is suggested.

Video

A video presentation of a group activity may then usefully demonstrate the social skills aspects with which we are concerned.

Questions

Finally a time for questions is offered. It is worthwhile for the therapist to be prepared for a variety of questions. In the main, she will not be required to have definitive answers, but be ready to elaborate on topics that have already arisen. Frequently, parents will ask for practical ideas as to how they can help, e.g. 'What should we actually do?' The therapist is able to explain that this will be fully addressed, in conjunction with the adolescent client, during the family session held during the second week of the course. At that time each client is given the opportunity to consider possible alternative strategies that each member of the family might adopt following the course.

Problem-solving

The parents then rejoin the adolescent group for the problem-solving activity which has been discussed earlier. (Note: appointments for family sessions may be made on this afternoon.)

Week 2

The essence of this week is to build on the foundational skills identified and practised during the first week. Clients will have finished the 'fluency factors' programme of communication skills and therapists will now encourage clients to employ fluency factors as and when necessary and as independently as possible. If reminders are requested then clients will negotiate the type of reminder, the frequency and the consequences of being reminded. For example, it may be that a group member feels that his self-monitoring skills still need to be improved. He may request that therapists only remind him to monitor his speech by use of a hand signal, up to three times per session. He will then self-reinforce if he is successful. Therapists will be aiming to reduce this to a minimum so that the choice of using fluency factors is wholly the client's.

Commonly, therapists have some difficulty in fulfilling this task. The instinct to offer advice and guidance is strong, however, the course is specifically designed to establish with the client that there are choices available and to practise these in the relative safety of the group setting. The client who does not take personal responsibility for experimentation will not transfer the newfound skills into the real world.

Emphasis then continues to be given to the broad area of communication skills during this second week. Further activities are offered to enhance listening, observation, turntaking, praise, self-reinforcement, problem-solving and negotiation. Videotape recordings are especially valuable in providing instant feedback for self-evaluation and constructive criticism of progress. The programme evolves towards providing opportunities for individuals, through role rehearsal and role play, to practise specific situations which they have identified as problematic.

The structure of the day is maintained as before with homework feedback, topic identification, activities and discussion.

Day 6

Following home work feedback, a revision of the previous week's aims is important to re-establish those aspects which are inherent in all activities and the features which may still need to be highlighted.

Fluency factors are now incorporated into group activities and each individual will be asked to decide whether reminders or further instruction is needed as identified above. It can be helpful to have personal aims for the day displayed on wall charts or white boards. These could

DAY SIX

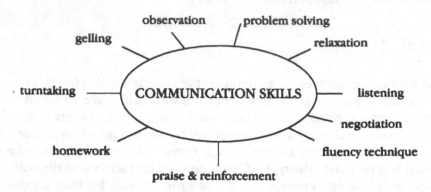

AM

10 . 00 GROUP GELLING ACTIVITY:
"The Name Came "

10.10 Homework Feedback in small groups -
nominate spokesperson to feedback to main
group - collect in difficult speaking situations

10.20 GROUP DISCUSSION:
Review of last week - What did you learn?
"What did you need more of? "

10.30 Fluency practice/relaxation

10.45 GROUP ACTIVITY:
"The Pink Elephant"

11.15 GROUP FLUENCY ACTIVITY
" Build a Story "

11.30 Review Negotiation Exercise: Desert Island
Exercise on Video
Re-Rate yourself on Social Skills Rating Scale

11.45 GROUP ACTIVITY:
Preparation for One Minute Video:
Reading Fluently in front of group

12.00 LUNCH TIME TASK:
i) Buy something in shop using fluency
factors to help you to be as fluent as possible
ii) Prepare a presentaion to group in pm on
any topic to be videoed

FLUENCY PRACTICE

THINGS TO REMEMBER

P M

1 00 Feedback from Lunchtime

1.10 GROUP ACTIVITY:
" Tangle "

120 Relaxation session sitting on chairs

1.30 GROUP ACTIVITY:
Two minute Video Presentations

1.50 Review videos - Each individual to identify
what his/her targets are in terms of fluency
and social skills

2.10 GROUP ACTIVITY:
" Ladders " Active game,
(listening)

2.25 GROUP ACTIVITY:
" The Balloon Debate " - (Turn Taking,
Negotiation, Assertiveness)

2.45 GROUP ACTIVITY:
Role Rehearsal e.g: Asking Directions

3.00 Good news/bad news
Homework:
i) Fluency task - asking for something in a
shop, asking directions
ii) Observation task - observe others rate of
speech—fast/slow

FLUENCY PRACTICE

THINGS TO REMEMBER

Figure 5.6 The communication skills approach: day 6

describe fluency factors, reminders, and other social skill aims. The videotape recordings from the previous week will serve as baseline samples.

Activities within the group, with their aims and objectives are, as usual, fully discussed.

Lunchtime tasks become progressively more demanding. It is essential to establish the transfer of skills outside the clinical setting at the earliest moment. The therapist's role is affirming the positive results. Another hidden trap awaits the unwary therapist! Despite consistency in avoiding emphasis on normal fluency as an objective for inside and outside assignments, it may still be the first response in the feedback sessions: *'My fluency broke down'*; *'I just couldn't get my technique to work'*, etc., etc. It is imperative to look for the 'good news' first! (e.g. they had a go; approached the situation thoughtfully; planned the activity; used appropriate eye-contact; tried not to rush, etc., etc.). Fluency is not the issue, after all they are accustomed to stuttering, and the focus on the new skills is more important. The expertise of the therapist is paramount in this respect.

The afternoon session continues with activities including debates, negotiation sessions and role rehearsal. Following each, the debriefing session identifies progress and offers openings for self-reinforcement.

Homework tasks are assigned to the group but may now be varying between individuals because of specific needs.

Day 7

Following homework feedback and discussion another dimension is introduced via the brainstorm technique: 'the advantages and disadvantages of speech techniques'.

It is well documented that clinical fluency is commonly quite accessible, however, it has also been demonstrated that the transfer of this fluency is extremely difficult. (See p. 60.) This activity seeks to explore those issues which are involved in the use of speech modification strategies and why they should only be seen as useful adjuncts, but not the whole answer to stuttering. The outcome of this exercise should help clients recognise that fluency factors, because they require a great deal of hard work, must become a matter of personal choice and may not always be an immediate option.

Discussion of speaking situations sets the agenda for the afternoon sessions. Assignments should be practised in a role play format within the clinic, and then introduced within the behavioural format of small incremental steps, building up towards real life practice. Commonly, early situations include asking directions, requesting information, making enquiries, asking the time. It is useful to re-look at the individual PQRST assessments, as these will identify particular personal situations.

DAY SEVEN

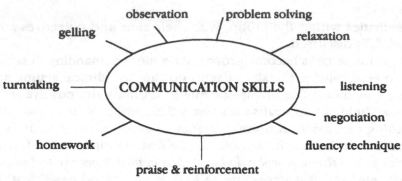

AM

10.00 GROUP ACTIVITY:
       " Fruit Salad "

10.10 Homework feedback

10.25 GROUP FLUENCY ACTIVITY:
       " The Yes/No Game "

10.45 BRAINSTORM:
       " The Advantages and Disadvantages of
       Technique";

11.00 Individual Fluency Practice/relaxation
       Make up own personal fluency/communica-
       tion plan

11.20 ROLE PLAY:
       Difficult speaking situations (Video)

11.45 GROUP DISCUSSION:
       Feedback on above exercise
       Outline plan for this pm

11.55 Lunchtime task:
       Asking for something in a shop - pair up and
       observe each other in light of individual
       fluency plans formulated today

PM

1.00   ASSIGNMENTS:
       Afternoon spent on telephone assignments:
       in pairs/triads with therapist allocated to
       each group

2.30   Re-convene group: Feedback from each
       individual

2.50   Good news/bad news
       Homework:
       i) Take each others telephone numbers and
       make at least two short telephone calls to
       other clients this evening.
       ii) Make one short practice telephone call to
       a friend or establishment

ASSIGNMENTS

THINGS TO REMEMBER

Figure 5.7 The communication skills approach: day 7

Pacing of these practical experiences is all-important. The clients will
need to know each stage in detail, the practice set up immediately and
the time constraint identified. This ascertains that no time is allowed for
the 'What if ...' problems. Calmness and expectation of success from the
therapist will be reassuring and will elicit trust. Following each step the
therapist asks for feedback and, as ever, looks for the good news.

Homework: additional assignments may be given, or the completion
of those outstanding from this day.

Day 8

As well as monitoring the structure of the day for the whole group, the therapists will need to focus on the family sessions which were organised on Day 5. It is recommended that an hour is set aside for a family session, although this will depend on the needs and size of the family. (See Appendix XVII for an outline of the family session and an example from a recent course). When the negotiation is completed, the therapist should record verbatim the agreements that have been made in the form of a contract. This is sent home with the family and a copy kept for the follow up meeting.

The morning session is structured as before but with increasingly demanding tasks and more emphasis on personal plans for the day. The therapists continue to encourage clients to take personal responsibility for their communication skills, and at all stages make use of opportunities to elicit evaluations and self-reinforcement of progress. The afternoon session is planned by the group during the morning and is contingent on previous assignments and their personal needs.

Role play is an important feature of the day. This could be of interview situations, or oral presentations, depending on the clients' needs.

Group activities which focus on fluency factors are still interspersed to ensure the continued understanding of the choices the client has available.

Day 9

The usual structure is in place, homework feedback as an essential first step and the ensuing discussion forming the basis for the assignments planned for the afternoon.

A brainstorm entitled **'The Advantages and Disadvantages of Stuttering'** is always of great interest and the focus of considerable controversy. The rationale behind this exercise is important: for some the increase in confidence and ability to communicate may have implications which can be construed negatively. At this point, clients may identify that they may lose certain concessions, e.g. be required to participate more fully than ever before in school as well as socially and at home.

Outside assignments are targeted on an individual basis, but commonly the clients pair up to achieve them. The mutual support and trust acquired over the course amongst the participants is now plain to see. All will be skilled in identifying the good news and reinforcing successes.

Day 10

The therapists' task today is to set the scene for what will happen after

DAY EIGHT

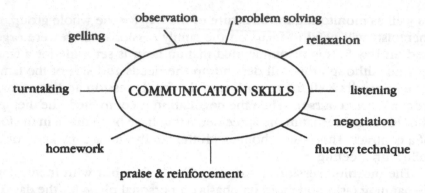

AM

10. 00 GROUP ACTIVITY:
        " Statues"

10.10   Homework feedback~
        Telephone calls

10.25   Prepare a piece of reading or monologue for
        3 minutes in front of main group to be
        videoed

10.30   GROUP ACTIVITY:
        Video Presentations

11.00   GROUP DEBATE:
        " How should schools help stammering
        pupils? "
        –turn taking,
        –problem solving,
        –assertion

11.20   GROUP FLUENCY ACTIVITY
        " Just a Minute "
        –interruption
        –assertion
        –fluency

11.35   GROUP ACTIVITY:
        " Stand on my Right "
        –assertion

11.50   Prepare precis for interview role play this
        pm

12.00   Lunchtime task:
        Pair up and ask for each other's lunch in
        shop, fluently

PM

1 . 00 GROUP ACTIVITY:

        ROLE PLAY: INTERVIEWS

2.00   Feedback from group and identify targets for
        improvement to try again tomorrow

2. 15   GROUP ACTIVITY:
        " Who am I ? "

2 . 3 5 GROUP ACTIVITY:
        " Describe a diagram "

2.45   ASSIGNMENTS:
        Paired with therapists to buy/cost items from
        local shops

3.00   Return to base: Feedback
        Homework:
         i) Fluency Task
         ii) Plan further assignments for tomorrow

3.15   Good news/bad news

ASSIGNMENTS

THINGS TO REMEMBER

Figure 5.8 The communication skills approach: day 8

DAY NINE

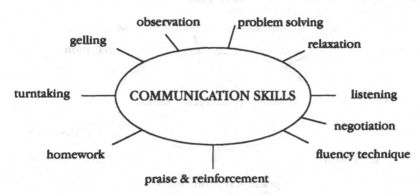

COMMUNICATION SKILLS

observation • problem solving • relaxation • gelling • turntaking • listening • negotiation • homework • fluency technique • praise & reinforcement

10.00 GROUP ACTIVITY:
" Land, Sea, Sky "

10.10 Homework feedback

10.20 BRAINSTORM:
"Advantages and Disadvantages of Stuttering"

10.30 Decide individual Targets for Today for:
i) Role Play
ii) Assignments
from yesterday's homework

10.40 Role plays and assignments

1 1.40 Return to base: Feedback on assignments
and role plays

11.55 Lunchtime tasks:
i) Plan further assignments form PQRST

Targets for Today
ii) Pair up and buy lunch for each other
using fluency factors

1.00 Lunchtime task feedback

1.15 GROUP FLUENCY ACTIVITY:
I went on holiday and I went to....."
(Rule game: Observation and Listening)

1.30 Assignments (including telephone practice)

2.35 Return to base: Feedback from assignments

2.55 Homework:
i) Practice Fluency Targets

ASSIGNMENTS

THINGS TO REMEMBER

Figure 5.9 The communication skills approach: day 9

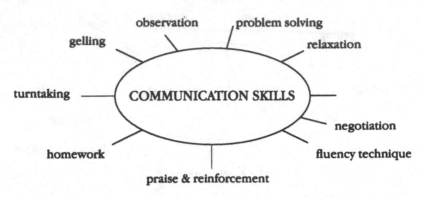

DAY TEN

AM

10.00   GROUP ACTIVITY:
        "Ladders "

10   Homework Feedback

10.30   BRAINSTORM:
        " What will I do if I become dysfluent? "

10.50   Individual final day assessments begin
        GROUP ACTIVITIES:
        " Call my Bluff "
        " Who am I? "

11.50   WHOLE GROUP ACTIVITY:
        Plan for future therapy needs
        Plan follow up appointments

12.00   Assignments : Go to buy lunch for group

12.30   Group Lunch
2.30   Farewells and exchange of addresses

Figure 5.10 The communication skills approach: day 10

the course. It is very likely that the group will feel very 'high' on their newfound skills and insight. Their confidence is at its greatest but it is very tenuous.

It is therefore important that the group considers the problems which may arise on their return to normal life and ordinary routines. It may be that individual members of the group will not have disclosed their attendance on the course to teachers or to peers, whereas others may have shared this information. Whatever the position, the therapist's role is to direct the group members' attention to potential scenarios and possible actions that can be taken. It may well be in the client's best interest to affirm that problems will occur.

Small group discussions focusing on likely pitfalls can be used to lead into a final brainstorm of 'How to Deal with Difficult Situations'. The ideas from this can be entered into the final page of the workbook and will be useful as revision or to development a self-help programme following the course.

This may be seen as putting a bit of a dampener on the last day of the course, but nonetheless predicting problems is realistic.

Final day assessments are completed. Follow up appointments are organised. Telephone numbers are exchanged. Programme books checked to ensure that clients take home their record of the course and particularly the final 'How to Deal ...?' brainstorm. A handout reviewing the course is also distributed. (Appendix XVIII).

The last assignment for the group is to organise lunch for the whole group including therapists!

Chapter 6
Environmental Influences

The focus of this chapter will be to consider those environmental factors which exert an influence upon the adolescent who stutters and may be compounding the problem. These include the changing nature of the adolescent–parent relationship, as well as the adolescent in the context of school, both in terms of relationships with authority figures and with peer groups. The role of the speech and language clinician is discussed.

Family involvement

In Chapter 2, the full assessment procedure was described which includes the separate interviews for the adolescent and parents. Both parents, where applicable, are involved in this process, with equal weight given to their observations and views and to those of the adolescent. The primary objective of this protocol is to formulate a composite picture of the adolescent and to gain an understanding of the dynamics of the individual family. From this information, the speech and language clinician can develop an hypothesis regarding environmental factors within the family which may be influencing or reinforcing the dysfluency. There are often indications that, as with other age groups, the family may need to be drawn into the therapeutic process in order to achieve positive change. Periodically, therefore, the speech and language therapist will identify issues within a family which require direct intervention because of their relevance to the maintenance of the stuttering.

The parents or adolescent may request help openly or indicate that there are difficulties within the relationship about which they are concerned but feel impotent. The decision to involve some or all of the family may be made following the initial interview, or at any stage during the therapy process. It may be necessary to work with the young adult on his own in the initial stages, as he may be antagonistic to the idea of parental involvement and need to be persuaded of the benefits of a joint venture.

In certain circumstances it may also be advisable to include the siblings, or even grandparents in sessions. Family intervention is, however, not possible without the full cooperation of all parties.

The role of the speech and language therapist

It is our contention that the main aim of family intervention is to reinstate the 'lines of communication' between the parents and their teenager. As we have noted in preceding chapters, adolescence is a continuous process of change and these transitions have reverberations for the whole family. Parents may feel very fearful for their son or daughter within society. The media focus on drugs, violence, sexual freedom, unemployment, etc. presents an outside world of inherent risk. Parents are inevitably confused and worried and, as a result, may fail to adjust their parenting styles to the young adult's increasing need for independence within the family. This is particularly evident when the adolescent is seen as socially disadvantaged because of a communication problem.

Through observation of and discussion with the family, the therapist will learn about the parents' views on child-rearing practices, including discipline, rules, routines, flexibility and the focus of disputes. In general, the important elements of conflict revolve around a breakdown of communication.

The therapist, in the role of the professional 'outsider', can serve as a facilitator and catalyst for the family. The skill of the therapist lies in the professional ability to conceptualise the problems in the context of the family's lifestyle and to suspend judgments which may emanate from personal experience. As identified in previous chapters, the therapist's art is in refraining from offering ideas or direct advice but in reframing the problem, encouraging alternative, positive ideas and then, by 'throwing the ball back into their court', permitting the family to find their own solutions.

Initially, less contentious issues can be addressed and, as the family develops the ability to empathise with each others' perceptions of the problem, more sensitive areas can be confronted.

By way of illustration, we present a case study of a 16-year-old girl and her family where direct family intervention was indicated.

Case study

'Jane was an only child of professional parents. During the initial family session it was noted that frequent intrusive interruptions were occurring from mother whilst father was speaking, something which was also observed in her communications with her daughter. Furthermore, mother adopted a steadfastly negative attitude about her daughter's speech problem, feeling that, if only she made more of an effort, she could be fluent. In her view Jane's main problem was that she was 'lazy, like her father'.'

'For his part, father had a more sympathetic view of his daughter's condition. However, it was difficult for the interviewer to keep father on track, as he frequently diverted from the topic, often adopting an accusative stance in relationship to his wife, who became more defensive as the interview progressed.'

'During subsequent video observation sessions, when the family was given a simple problem-solving exercise, father was often observed to allow his daughter to use him as her 'mouthpiece' when communicating and, in particular, if there was any friction between herself and her mother, she would rely on her father to speak for her.'

'Jane was prone to episodes of silent sulking when she did not get her own way, and was characterised by her mother as an 'uncommunicative child'.'

'There was inconsistency in the discipline regimes employed by mother and father. Mother was rather inflexible in her approach, whereas father was likely to 'say one thing and do another' after persistent nagging by his daughter.'

'The speech and language clinician felt that the communication styles within the family were a major contributor to the maintenance of Jane's moderate dysfluency and associated avoidance strategies. It was clear that the communicative behaviour was to a large extent the manifestation of underlying tensions within the triad which needed to be resolved.'

'In essence the focus of the intervention was to:

1. Develop mother and father's understanding of the nature of stuttering.
2. Explore more productive communication skills in relationship to each other, including turntaking, with the aim of reducing conflict.
3. Teach the parents more effective strategies in the reinforcement of positive behaviours.'

'Jane was also taught more effective communication styles, including active listening, negotiation and problem-solving skills.'

Jane's parents were not the cause of her stuttering behaviour, but there was strong evidence to suggest that some of their own behaviours were influencing and compounding the problem.

Child-rearing styles

Zarb (1992) proposes a model for the identification of 'dysfunctional child-rearing styles' which provides a useful framework for the identification of potential sources of tension which could pose significant barriers to effective treatment. (See Table 6.1.)

It is recognised that the speech and language clinician's remit will only enable him or her to offer direct support for those aspects of the family's communication styles which:

• Will be responsive to the interventions which she can offer.
• The family is motivated to change.

Where these two factors are not present, onward referral to more appropriate agencies is the recommended option.

During the next section of this chapter, we consider the possible range of direct interventions which might be offered by the speech and language clinician to the families of adolescents who stutter.

Family interventions

Epstein, Schlesinger and Dryden (1988) suggest that family sessions, mediated by a clinician, provide a useful forum for family members to express their views about each other and for these perceptions to be questioned by others within the family, where appropriate. Mutual perceptions can thus be evaluated and reconsidered.

Many professionals believe that effective family therapy can only be carried out within whole family sessions. This may not be feasible or appropriate in many situations. We have found that some parents are initially resistant to family sessions and may consider that the responsibility for the problem lies entirely with the adolescent. For example, in the third case history presented in Chapter 3, Lisa's mother found it hard to accept that she had any part to play in what was her daughter's problem and could not see why it should be necessary for her to be involved in the therapeutic process.

In order to establish a relationship of trust from the outset, the parents and client need to be convinced by the therapist that she empathises with each of their respective points of view.

In situations where there is conflict between parties, this sense of trust may more easily be accomplished by individual sessions with the parents and the adolescent before the combined sessions. Equally, there may be a case for two therapists to be allocated to a family: one working with the adolescent, the other simultaneously with the parents. We have used both of these models in our own clinic and have found them highly effective.

There are a number of circumstances where the role of the speech and language therapist is limited. For example, where parental conflict arises from a serious underlying dysfunction within the marriage, it can be most effective to recommend concurrent marital therapy, or there may be alcohol-related problems which, again, require onward referral.

In a small number of recent cases, young adults have been referred where suicide has been attempted with stuttering identified as the cause. Clearly, in such cases, psychotherapy would be indicated in the first instance with speech and language therapy offered as an important resource as soon as possible.

Parent-centred sessions

The object of parent-centred sessions is to explore alternative management strategies. These sessions intentionally comprise the therapist and

Table 6.1 Model of 'dysfunctional child-rearing styles' (Zarb, 1992)

Parental child-rearing style	Adolescent's habitual response
Punitive	
• physical/verbal aggression	• seeks retaliation
• punitive, guilt engendering	• self-punishment
	• extreme guilt
	• approval-seeking
	• adopts victim role
	• fearful obedience
Rejecting	
• adolescent unacceptable	• approval-seeking with parents,
• lacks affection for child	peers and others
	• excessive demands, tests limits
	• easily offended
	• suspicious of others
	• conduct disorder
Overcoercion	
• excessive parental control	• dependent on others for direction
• excessive parental nagging	• active resistance
	• passive resistance
	• lacks persistence, irresponsible
Overindulgence	
• overprotection	• bored passivity
• low expectations for child	• abdicates responsibility
	• lacks persistence: irresponsible
	• manipulates others
Oversubmissive	
• unable to set limits	• impulsive response style
• submits to adolescent's manipulations	• seeks immediate gratification
	• conduct disorder
	• self-destructive behaviour
	• lacks persistence; irresponsible
	• manipulative
Neglecting	
(due to illness, alcoholism, separation,	• avoids forming close relationships
death, desertion)	• lacks empathy
	• social skills deficit
	• makes excessive demands
	• depression
	• pre-occupied with parental neglect
	• excessive striving
	• manipulative
	• self-blame
	• drifting
Perfectionistic	
• demands excellence	• excessive striving
• withholds approval	• self-belittlement
	• guilt
Parental hypochondriasis	
	• uses illness as an excuse for avoidance
	• failure to take responsibility
	• performance anxiety

both parents without the adolescent present. The effectiveness of later combined sessions is enhanced if parents have had the previous opportunity to explore different behaviours and practise new strategies.

The use of videotape recording during these sessions is beneficial as it provides instant feedback. This promotes greater objectivity about current skills and, therefore, offers parents the opportunity to identify areas which may benefit from a different approach.

Separate sessions also provide the opening for the therapist to identify and question any negative attitudes or beliefs. Exploration of these will enable the parents to reconstrue certain aspects of the adolescent's behaviour. This also promotes positive change in management techniques.

Case study

One example of this was Timothy, aged 17, whose mother was becoming increasingly irritated by his 'silences' during mealtimes. She felt that he was being *deliberately uncommunicative and unresponsive* to *'even the most ordinary questions'*. Timothy's father agreed with his wife to some extent, but added that since the two sisters and Mother were *'always talking, it was quite hard for a chap to compete!'*

'The aim of the therapist here was to gain more information about the general patterns of turntaking within the family. This was achieved by setting a homework task whereby the mother and father, separately, observed the family at mealtimes to decide who did the most (a) talking, (b) interrupting and (c) listening. This first task set the scene for a continued discussion about the opportunities for entering conversations, the topic of the conversations and the rate of the interchanges.'

'Meanwhile in a separate session, Timothy was well aware of his mother's complaint, saying in the first instance that *'they were lucky he bothered to turn up to mealtimes, they were so boring!'*. He was given the same observation task concerning talking, interrupting and listening.'

'The outcome of this simple exercise was that Timothy's mother understood that it was very hard for him to compete on an equal basis partly because of the stuttering, but more importantly because he was not and never would be a 'chatterer', preferring the 'listener role' in this situation. Indeed, as the discussion progressed, both parents remembered comments by friends complaining of 'moodiness and sullen silence' in their own adolescents' behaviour, which was usually blamed on this adolescent 'phase of life'!'

'Father discovered that although he had agreed initially with his wife about Timothy, he was not a great contributer either—which he attributed to the 'female' topics of conversation! Mother learned that while she talked enthusiastically, and asked lots of questions, she seldom listened to the whole reply. Timothy realised that his lack of contribution to conversations might explain why the topics held little interest for him, and that by taking a more active role he could introduce new subjects. Possible turntaking rules were discussed and agreed changes implemented.'

These on-going sessions create an open forum for parents to discuss their attempts at instituting newly developed management strategies and to identify successes and difficulties which arise. This allows them to reframe each experience and to decide together how to tackle similar situations in the future. It can also be beneficial to ask parents to reflect on memories of their own adolescence and the relationship with their parents; similarities to the current situation can often be recalled.

During such sessions the parents' motivation and capacity for change will become evident, as well as their abilities to problem-solve together.

As described above, the adolescent will be participating in separate, perhaps concurrent sessions, and it is important to coordinate the phases of intervention for mutual benefit.

The success of such intervention is dependent upon the therapist being open and explicit with the family about the purpose of the intervention. Thus a sense of partnership will be established with a common aim of resolving areas of stress or tension within the family relationships.

Zarb (1992) provides a helpful summary of the important points which should be communicated to parents before implementation of a parent-centred programme and we have adapted these to reflect the special focus on stuttering behaviour in adolescents:

- The parents' responsibility is primarily to assist the adolescent to become a competent, well adjusted, independent and responsible individual. This may require a change in their own approach to handling the adolescent and his stuttering behaviour.
- Parents can learn more productive parenting and management strategies in relation to the adolescent's current problems, including his stuttering behaviour.
- Positive attitude and belief on the part of parents can produce more effective parenting styles and reduce conflict between parents and their adolescent.
- Whilst parents are expected to exert greater patience than would be expected of an adolescent, this does not mean that the son or daughter should be allowed to manipulate them.
- Both parents and teenager will be expected to negotiate and compromise.
- The dynamics of families mean that one member's behaviour will have an effect on another's behaviour.
- The adolescent's problem (i.e. stuttering) is a joint family problem, and the quality of interactions between the adolescent, parents and other family members will function either to maintain or reduce the problematic behaviour.

The therapist needs to take into account the strengths and weaknesses of each parent as well as their ability to work together, in order to plan a programme of training which is realistic and achievable.

Stategies for intervention

Cognitive restructuring

This technique is central to family interventions and is aimed at enabling family members to recognise and re-evaluate attitudes, beliefs and expectations of each other which are irrational or unrealistic. Misperceptions occur because an individual pays selective attention to information (i.e. notices certain aspects and overlooks others), opinions then become magnified over time (i.e 'blown up out of all proportion'), and this may lead to over-generalising (i.e making one observation apply to all situations) of the belief.

There are four steps in the process of restructuring biased beliefs or mistaken assumptions within the parent–adolescent relationship in order to reduce conflict:

1. Identification of the biased belief or mistaken assumption: this requires the therapist to reflect back those perceptions identified as being the source of the conflict.
2. Testing the logic behind the faulty opinion: through direct feedback, exaggeration, questioning, humour or reframing techniques, i.e. looking at the issue from a more positive perspective.
3. Encouraging alternative, more positive and flexible perceptions.
4. Prompting ideas for a solution which are consistent with the new, flexible perception and inviting the family to experiment with this, initially through rehearsal, then in reality, to see whether this is successful.

Case study

'Following the recent separation of his parents, David, aged 15, and his brother, aged 17, had recently set up home together with their father. Family sessions with David and his father had been arranged because of the rapidly escalating disputes between them about eating, bedtime and studying. These were clearly having a detrimental effect on David's stuttering.'

'David reported to the therapist that he was *always* hungry when he got in from school and there was *never* anything in the house to eat and that his father *continuously* nagged him about his late hours and lack of study.'

'Father said that he was struggling to keep the fridge full, could not believe how often he had to shop for food for the two boys and they *never* forewarned him when stocks were low. In addition he was very worried that David was out late *every* night with friends, was *always* tired in the morning and was doing *no* school work *at all*.'

This information was imparted to the therapist who, while asking each for clarification of their individual perceptions, made sure that all statements were made directly to her.

The first topic to be discussed concerned the supply of and demand for food. This was deemed a relatively non-contentious issue and, following the initial disclosures regarding their own points of view, each was invited to describe his understanding of the other person's position. The therapist then identified and explored the area of conflict, reflected this back and, by focusing on the 'selective attention', the 'magnification' and the 'over-generalisation' on each side (i.e. 'always', 'never', 'continuously', etc), was able to reframe the distorted opinions. The therapist was then able to prompt new ideas for discussion and possible implementation.

The outcome was that David achieved a greater understanding of his father's difficult new role as housekeeper while father, in turn, discovered that adolescents have voracious appetites which might be relieved by joint forward planning.

Each area of contention was dealt with in a similar way: David learned to understand his father's perceptions and fears while his father understood that 'nagging' was not the best way forward and that by reducing his need to direct and control, David would have to take responsibility for his own mistakes, i.e. being late for school through tiredness and failing exams because of insufficient study.

Patterns of interactive communication within families

One of the most common complaints from the parents of our clients is that their teenager does not talk to them. However, although this may be ascribed to being 'just a phase', many parents do not recognise that this seeming reluctance may be due, in part, to their own lack of interactive skills.

As noted in previous chapters, successful interpersonal communication is dependent on a broad range of social skills (Rustin and Kuhr, 1989), including observation, listening, turntaking, praise and reinforcement, problem-solving and negotiation. These, therefore, can be the focus for assessing the communication styles within families.

The following checklist (Table 6.2) identifies, through behavioural analysis, problematic interactions which could be contributing to the maintenance of stuttering and proposes alternative, more constructive, strategies.

The following procedures have been found useful in identifying areas for modification.

Homework observation tasks

Aspects of each of the social skills components can be probed through home-based observations. For example, each member of the family is instructed to observe whether praise is given within their household. A homework sheet is given to record when an individual has given any praise, what was said and how it was received. This is done independently and with no collaboration. This requires members to make objective observations of the interactions of various family members. The information brought back to sessions can be used for discussion on the value of praise, its quality and frequency. (See Chapter 4, p. 67.)

Other home-based observation tasks can be given, which focus on the listening skills and the patterns of turntaking commonly used within the family, as well as the opportunities for mutual problem-solving and negotiation between members.

In addition, a videotape recording of the family working together to solve a problem or negotiate an issue in the clinical setting, offers the therapist direct observation of the family's interaction. The family group can suggest simple problems of their own or the therapist may be able to offer suggestions which are pertinent. The checklist (Table 6.2) for identifying patterns of interaction can then be completed.

The instant feedback of videotape recording is a remarkably effective technique for enabling family members to identify areas for change and opportunities to develop self-help strategies.

If necessary the therapist can propose alternative strategies and model these to the family. Family members can then experiment with these during a role rehearsal activity within the family session.

Problem-solving training

This is an effective skills training approach which may be applied to both individual family members, dyads, triads or families as a whole. Rustin (1987) and Mallard (1991) have outlined a family approach to problem-solving which has direct relevance to the adolescent who stutters:

*   Problem definition.
*   Generation of alternative solutions.
*   Decision-making.
*   Planning solution implementation.

The first task is to identify which member of the family has an appropriate problem which they could share, and whether the rest of the family would be willing to help. The problem definition phase is then important. With an adolescent, for example, this might be concerned with 'failure to complete homework' or 'getting into trouble through not letting parents know his whereabouts' or 'getting up late in the mornings', etc. The adolescent is encouraged to be explicit about his view of the problem. He should be prompted to describe the specific circumstances and his consequent feelings until all feel that they have a clear understanding from the perspective of the 'problem-holder'.

The problem, explicitly defined, is written on a sheet of paper which

Table 6.2 Parent–adolescent interaction checklist

Problematic behaviours	Alternative behaviours
rapid speech rate	slower speech rate
overuse of questions	reduce questions, use of comments, statements, etc.
poor listening	active listening, maintaining conversation, reflecting, acknowledging, following topic
interrupting	active listening, awareness of conversation turns
lack of reinforcement	use of non-verbal and verbal cues, e.g. nodding, agreement
monopolising	briefer statement, response time latency, tolerance of silence, pausing
commanding, overdirective	negotiating, suggesting alternatives, seeking other ideas, views
inappropriate body language	awareness of eye-contact, posture, distance, gesture, mannerisms

all can see. The family members, including the adolescent, now generate a range of possible solutions which are also recorded. At this stage, no comment should be allowed about the relative merits of the suggestions—all should be recorded, until no more are forthcoming. At this point the problem-holder is asked to decide which possible solutions are acceptable and which are unacceptable. He is asked to rationalise his decisions, giving reasons why he is rejecting solutions and this is discussed by the whole family. A minimum of three acceptable solutions should be identified which can then be rank ordered in terms of preference.

The final phase involves a joint plan between family members as to how the solutions can be implemented with their support. The family and the therapist then reach an agreement about monitoring, evaluation and feedback mechanisms.

Case study

'Jim, aged 17, identified a problem with budgeting his allowance. By the end of each month he was consistently in debt to both friends and family, although the amount he was getting was deemed to be adequate and reasonable. This problem was used during a family session comprising Jim, both parents and an older brother, to institute better problem-solving skills. The problem was defined as 'Jim's difficulty with budgeting his allowance'. The family then generated 25 possible alternative solutions which were recorded verbatim. Jim then considered each possibility, discarded a number as impractical, unattainable, impossible, unthinkable, etc. and finally had a hierarchy of four possible solutions. Jim's first choice was to sub-divide the allowance into a daily rate, trying to save a small proportion of this for a weekly binge!'

Clearly, it may not always be a problem related specifically to the adolescent which is considered. Indeed, it is more beneficial if problems are not solely focused on the adolescent and he is involved in generating solutions for other family members.

The essence of this approach is that it encourages positive family dialogue, constructive criticism and a real sense of shared responsibility and mutual support which invariably proves highly reaffirming to the family unit.

Negotiation skills training

This is another effective strategy for family intervention when lines of communication have broken down. Kifer, Lewis, Green and Phillips (1974) encourage family members to use three types of verbal negotiation styles:

1. Complete communications—indicating one's own position in relation to the issue at hand and actively seeking the explicit position of other parties to the issue.
2. Statements which identify issues—that is, making statements which clearly identify the points of conflict and clarify the other parties' points of view.
3. Statements of options—these are statements which attempt to provide possible options and alternatives for productive solutions which will be acceptable to all parties.

Negotiation sessions follow on from the problem-solving training and initial tasks are carried out within the clinic.

In most instances, it is best to start with an issue for negotiation which is relatively non-emotive for the family.

The therapist's role is to model and direct family members to use those styles of exchange indicated above, until they have understood the basic principle of negotiation, which is that a mutually acceptable solution is reached. This may require adherence by all parties to one particular member's point of view or a compromise between family members' various standpoints. Again, video feedback can be used which allows the family to rehearse and refine negotiation skills through objective observation of their own performance.

Contingency contracting

Although this technique has largely been employed in relation to adolescents displaying conduct disorders, we have found that it adapts particularly well for use with families of adolescents who stutter. The notion of contingency contracting is that family members are asked, during a combined session, to identify behaviours that they would like another family member to adapt, in exchange for a reward for a successful change of that behaviour.

Once agreement has been reached, these changes form the basis of a contract between involved parties.

The most important element of a workable contract of this kind is explicitness; that is, all parties should understand clearly what their responsibilities are and what is expected of them, what the privileges and the penalties will be upon success or failure to bring about the agreed change in behaviour and an understanding that these will be carried through on a consistent basis.

The effectiveness of contingency contracting may be shown in the following case study.

Case study

'Ian, a 15-year-old, was disturbed by his father's persistent habit of attempting to finish his sentences for him during severe blocks. A contract was set up between Ian and his father in which Mr C agreed to stop this habit in return for the 'reward' that Ian would go fishing with him one weekend a month. However, the penalty, if he failed to comply with the terms of the contract and interrupted his son whilst he was stuttering, was that he would miss his monthly fishing trip (a pastime he valued beyond all others), and he would be obliged to take Ian ten-pin bowling instead, his son's favourite hobby.'

'Before the contract was formally signed, a session was agreed to explore Mr C's feelings of anxiety and frustration when his son stuttered and, with Ian's help, to reframe his perceptions of the situation. Alternative responses to the stuttering were thus agreed and practised.'

'The father's successes or failures to comply were monitored by both parties on a record chart, which outlined the date, time and nature of any interruptions. After 2 months the habit had ceased and Ian felt much happier about his communication exchanges with his father. Mr C reported that he was more relaxed about his son's stuttering and no longer felt the temptation to finish Ian's sentences.'

With a combination of cognitive restructuring, communication skills training and contingency contracting, Ian's father was able to sustain a change in an unproductive response pattern because he had a much clearer understanding of the negative impact of this behaviour upon his son.

It is important for the therapist to identify real motivators, to be clear about the methods by which the contract can be monitored, and to gain agreement to the terms from both parties.

Intervention within the school setting

The young adult functions in a variety of social milieux beyond the family unit and relationships with other significant groups assume an increasing importance in the adolescent's life as he develops into a social, independent and mature individual. Therefore, to gain a comprehensive picture of the adolescent who stutters and the demands of his world, some account should be taken of his school environment. For many young people, school life is a major source of tension.

The main task facing the speech and language therapist in this event is to enable the client to identify those aspects of school which are problematic and, from this information, to discriminate between those issues which could be responsive to therapeutic interventions within the clinic and those which may require constructive and practical alternative strategies within the school setting.

Teacher–adolescent relationships

The vast majority of teachers are understanding, sympathetic individuals who are motivated to do the best for students under their care. However, for many teachers, the disorder of stuttering can be bewildering and confusing when encountered in the classroom.

The role of the speech and language clinician in the school context is as an educator and facilitator of positive management change. In the general sense, it is important to provide schools with information and literature about practical classroom management strategies which will encourage, rather than inhibit, the young person's contribution. Teachers also need to be aware of the possible educational, psychological, emotional and behavioural impacts of a chronic stutter upon an individual, in terms of peer socialisation, teasing, bullying, associated learning difficulties, etc. It is important to share pertinent information with teachers about those components of the student's dysfluency and associated problems which will affect his educational and social welfare. This is best accomplished with the full cooperation and involvement of parents and adolescent to ensure a consistent approach. Where teacher–pupil conflict has arisen, it is usually the result of misunderstanding and a breakdown of communication. Teachers, like parents, will need space to discuss their perceptions of the student in an open forum. Where the speech and language clinician perceives inaccurate assumptions or beliefs about the individual and his communication difficulties, she will need to employ similar strategies to those outlined earlier in this chapter.

Thus, providing information on the nature and development of stuttering will enable teachers to re-evaluate their perceptions of the student and discussion of alternative management strategies may obviate occasions for conflict.

At a practical level, such interfacing between teachers and therapists invariably requires the therapist to visit the school environment. This experience can be invaluable as it gives the clinician a far greater insight into those school-related issues discussed during individual treatment sessions.

Case study

> 'Paul, a 15-year-old client had been on an intensive 2-week fluency
> programme during which his level of fluency had improved considerably.
> However, upon his return to school, he began to experience difficulties main-
> taining his new found fluency during two classes in particular, both of which
> were with teachers he 'did not like'. On further investigation it appeared that
> these two teachers were both aware of his attendance on the course, and as a
> result, had revised their expectations of Paul's fluency. Demands upon him
> during class activities had consequently risen, which had outstripped his
> tenuous hold on fluency. This engendered a negative reaction both from Paul
> and from his teachers. With the family's agreement, the speech and language
> clinician arranged a meeting to which the form tutor, the two teachers in
> question and other interested teachers were invited.'
>
> 'In the event, six teachers attended the meeting, during which the speech
> and language clinician explained the content of the intensive course in more
> detail and ascertained the staff's expectations of therapy. Through discussion,
> the therapist was able to revise the teachers' perceptions and to agree consis-
> tent and practical management strategies. In fact, as a result of the meeting
> the school developed an additional section to its special needs policy to
> incorporate recommended management principles in relation to students
> who stutter.'

Peer relationships

This represents another aspect of the environmental influences which
may need to be considered when working with adolescents who stutter.
It is important for the clinician to understand the peer network of the
client, the value systems which operate within it, and the resultant pressures. Although there is a risk of over-emphasising potential difficulties
for a client in terms of successful social integration with peers, many
adolescents who stutter have wide and varied social networks. However,
there does exist a small group for whom social integration has been a
problem. There may be numerous, complex reasons why a person has
failed to develop a range of social contacts, and initial consideration
might be given to the individual's social communication skills which
have been discussed previously. A framework for intervention on these
aspects will be found in chapters 4 and 5. However, some of the reasons
may realistically be beyond the control of the person himself and relate
more to a lack of acceptance within the local culture. It is essential that
the clinician recognises and explores such possibilities thoroughly in
order to avoid developing unrealistic or inappropriate expectations of
the client. In some ways, this presents more of a challenge to the clinician who is attempting to improve the opportunities for social integration of her client. In instances where there appears to be no obvious
social skills deficit on the part of the client, it may be valuable to obtain
more information from others in the adolescent's world, including the
family and teachers.

It may be that the clinician needs to employ some cognitive restructuring techniques, problem-solving and negotiation skills training with the young adult in order to encourage him to exert more positive influence over others and more effective response styles, thus enhancing the potential for positive peer relationships.

However, in rare circumstances it may be that a persistent, negative culture exists around the individual and it will be important to explore what realistic potential there is for change within the current environment and what would be required to bring this about. Alternative educational and social settings may also be considered by the clinician, client and his parents. It may fall to the speech and language clinician to suggest such changes and although it is recognised that such proposals will appear quite radical in nature, they may be the only way for the young person to develop to his full potential.

Case study

Gregory, a 15-year-old client with a moderate, intermittent stutter, referred himself back to our service during a phase when his dysfluency had become particularly severe. It transpired that he was the victim of increasingly aggressive taunts from two boys who attended his school. He felt helpless in dealing with these boys and had become increasingly isolated and resentful, as well as very dysfluent. A programme of problem-solving training and role play was implemented with Gregory, focusing on developing a wider repertoire of response styles to the taunts of his peers. The aim of this intervention was to increase his own sense of control in the situation, and to help him to appreciate that he could actively do something to improve the situation. However, the problem had become so established that it was necessary to make contact with Gregory's head of year to inform him of the situation. In collaboration, a plan of action was developed which included a negotiation/reconciliation session between Gregory and his antagonists, led by the head of year, and a workshop presentation to be organised for Gregory's year group. The focus of this workshop was to be communication, with a particular emphasis on the experiences of those who have a communication difficulty. This session, with Gregory's consent, was to be run jointly by the speech and language therapist and the head of year. In the event, the negotiation session was so successful in resolving the problem between Gregory and the two boys that further assistance was not required. Above all, he felt in a stronger position to deal with any subsequent teasing in a more assertive, positive style.

Environmental influences play an important part in the successful management of stuttering in adolescence. The speech and language therapist has the opportunity to play a central role in facilitating productive and positive changes for both the client and significant others in his world.

Whilst we in no way pretend that the areas of identification and remediation of environmental influences upon the adolescent stutterer present straightforward or simple tasks to the speech and language clinician, we feel that helpful structures do exist and, indeed, can be further developed to allow for the objective examination of those influences in order to inform appropriate intervention strategies. Furthermore, we do believe that our experience and knowledge as speech and language clinicians enables us to make valuable contributions to this vital component in the comprehensive management of the adolescent stutterer, which can result in productive and positive change for both the client and those significant others in his world.

Chapter 7
Language Impairment and the Adolescent Who Stutters

Claire Topping, B. Med. Sci. (Speech)

Principal Speech and Language Therapist for Mainstream Schools and Language Impairments, Camden and Islington Community Health Services (NHS) Trust.

The search for a conclusive link between language impairment (a specific and significant delay in expressive and/or receptive language, without sensory, cognitive or emotional impairment) and stuttering has been extensive and is well documented (Nippold, 1990; Bernstein Ratner, in press). Researchers have investigated the potential relationship of stuttering to acquisition of first words (e.g. Okasha et al., 1974; Seider, Gladstein and Kidd, 1982), syntax and morphology (e.g. Wall, 1980; Westby, 1974), semantics, (e.g. Williams, Melrose and Woods, 1969; Murray and Reed, 1977) and word finding ability (e.g. Boysen and Cullman, 1971).

Nippold (1990) summarises her review as follows:

> The view that stuttering children as a group, are more likely than non-stutterers to have delayed or disordered speech and language development has not been proven, despite more than 60 years of research. However, as some studies have reported speech and language delays or disorders in stutterers, clinicians should be alert to the possibility that any given child who stutters may have additional communication problems that warrant attention.
>
> (Nippold, 1990, p. 57).

Ehren (1994) identifies three subgroups of the adolescent population with language impairment:

1. A personal history which includes significant language impairment identified from an early age.
2. A history of academic difficulties not attributed to an underlying language impairment.
3. Language-related academic problems emerging only during adolescence.

The search to develop increasingly complex models of language processing is ongoing. The move is currently away from diagnostic labelling towards an integrated model which can account for a number

127

of manifestations of speech and language impairment within the same
system of analysis (e.g. Stackhouse and Wells, 1993). The concept of
working memory (Baddley and Hitch, 1974) is central to a number of
researchers' investigations. The role it plays in vocabulary acquisition,
speech production, reading development, skilled reading and language
comprehension has been explored by a number of researchers and
Baddley and Gathercole (1993) provide a comprehensive review of this
work. Lahey and Bloom (1994) use the notion of working memory in
conjunction with the concept of *mental models* (Johnson-Laird, 1983)
to present a model of capacity and demand which provides insight into a
range of phenomena relating to the performance of children with
language impairment. A mental model is defined as 'the representations
or momentary contents of consciousness that underlie intentional
actions and the interpretations of the actions of others' (Lahey and
Bloom, 1994, p. 356). As discussed in Chapter 1, Starkweather (1987)
developed a demand and capacity model of fluency development and
the possible links between these two models will now be explored.

Central to Lahey and Bloom's (1994) model is the notion of a limited
capacity system through which all information passes. Thus, both external perceptual information is processed and internal representations in
long-term memory retrieved to form mental models via working
memory. In addition to linguistic and cognitive information, social and
emotional demands are also processed within this limited capacity
system. If the sum of demands exceed the capacity, breakdown will
occur. However, the precise point of breakdown will vary depending on
the particular constellation of demands at any given time. It is proposed
that one of the key ways of reducing the demand is the overlearning of
skills so that they can be executed at a subconscious level. The often-
used analogy of learning to drive a car demonstrates this well. Initially,
basic skills, such as changing gear, require conscious attention. Over
time this skill becomes 'automatic' and is completed without conscious
thought, freeing the person to concentrate on other aspects of driving. If
this process of 'automisation' (Lahey and Bloom, 1994) is slowed down,
acquisition of new skills will take longer and require greater amounts of
practice. It is well recognised that for children with either language
impairment or with a stutter, certain language tasks which appear to be
automatic for most people require conscious effort. Within this model it
is possible, therefore, to view fluency parameters as a component of the
total linguistic demands being placed on the system. This interpretation
is supported by research in stuttering which identifies the loci of dysfluency as occurring at specific and predictable linguistic boundaries, such
as utterance-initial and clause-initial words (Bernstein, 1981; Wall et al.,
1981; Wingate, 1976), and on the initial words of sentential
constituents, such as noun phrases, verb phrases and prepositional
phrases (Bernstein, 1981). It could be hypothesised that these points

represent instances of extensive linguistic demands being placed on the limited capacity system and when the capacity is exceeded, breakdown manifests as dysfluency. It could also be hypothesised that the co-occurrence of stuttering and language impairment may render some individuals vulnerable to long-term communication difficulties.

In addition to providing a theoretical framework, the adoption of a model of capacity and demand has significant implications for the management for both language impairment and stuttering. By accepting the tenet of a limited capacity system, the clinician is led to two possible intervention strategies:

1. Increase the effective use of the capacity available, i.e. the automisation of tasks, which can be achieved through overlearning, reduces the demands placed on the system. (See Lahey and Bloom (1994) for detailed explanation.)
2. Decrease the external demands being placed on the system, i.e. the modification of the demands of the environment so that the system can work effectively within its capacity without breakdown occurring.

Thus, it would be predicted that the development of specific language skills and strategies combined with a modification of the social and emotional demands placed on the system would lead to an increased likelihood of developing and maintaining fluency. If we return to Ehren's (1994) description of the three subgroups of adolescents with language impairment, the model outlined above provides a possible explanation for the existence of the third group, that is the group whose language impairment only becomes apparent in adolescence. The requirement for increasing complexity in written language in secondary school is well documented, for example the shift from a narrative to a range of expository styles of text (Scott, 1994). This could be interpreted as an increased linguistic demand on a previously balanced system and represents the proverbial 'straw that breaks the camel's back' and results in language-related difficulties.

Assessment of language skills

There are two aspects to the assessment of language skills in adolescents who stutter. Firstly, the possible detection of a previously unidentified language disorder and, secondly, to aid the differential diagnosis of behaviours which may be attributable to either stuttering or language impairment or a combination of the two.

Identification of a language impairment

In a similar way to younger children, an adolescent person may experience difficulties in any aspect of language. It is the manifestation of those difficulties that will be qualitatively different. As a child develops it is the ability to integrate a range of both language and cognitive skills to complete increasingly complex tasks, such as reading and writing, which is needed. High-level difficulties in component skills may become compounded when those skills require integration. Assessment of language skills within this context requires the careful analysis of difficulties experienced in complex tasks so that key skills can be identified and an appropriate intervention programme planned.

Ehren (1994, pp. 396–397) provides a useful summary of the most common language characteristics which may be evident in both the spoken and written language of adolescents with language impairment. She identifies six key areas:

1. Word meaning and relationship difficulties, e.g. gaps in vocabulary, difficulty defining words, interpreting words with multiple meanings.
2. Word structure, e.g. lack of morphological markers in written language, imprecise use of word forms, poor discrimination of speech sounds.
3. Word retrieval, e.g. use of non-specific vocabulary, circumlocution.
4. Phrase structure, e.g. inability to make predictions, inaccurate interpretation of discourse.
5. Sentence structure, e.g. difficulty with the interpretation and expression of complex ideas.
6. Discourse/text, e.g. lack of flexibility in interpretation, difficulty synthesising information to obtain the central message.

In order to identify the presence of a language impairment information needs to be gathered from a wide range of sources and Klein (1985) provides a detailed assessment framework for older children and adolescents' spoken language skills.

Use of standardised tests

Clearly, standardised test materials provide useful information about the performance of any individual in comparison with peers of the same age. The limitations of formal tests are well known, particularly in relation to how well the demands of the test relate to real life situations. However, the initial identification of a language impairment is helped by the use of such measures. There is a range of formal tests available and some these are briefly discussed below.

The British Picture Vocabulary Scale (Dunn et al., 1982)

Age range: 2;11–18;1. A test of receptive vocabulary, it is available in a short form for rapid screening and long form for more detailed investigation.

Clinical Evaluation of Language Fundamentals—Revised Screening Test (Semel, Wiig and Secord, 1989)

Age range: 5;0–16;0. A basic test with a pass/fail criterion, it also contains a useful supplementary section for evaluating written language via the interpretation and recall of a short story. It has additional stories available for retest situations. The following areas are assessed: story organisation, detail and elaboration, sentence structure, maintenance of meaning and writing mechanics.

Clinical Evaluation of Language Fundamentals—Revised (Semel, Wiig and Secord, 1987)

Age range: 5;0–16;0. This test provides a total language score which gives an age equivalent rating. This score can be broken down for comparison into receptive and expressive language values. Performance on individual subtests can also be compared. Several of the subtests involve reading and there is the facility to substitute alternative tests and still yield a total language score where reading difficulties are known to exist. The test was originally standardised on an American population and a UK edition (Klein et al., 1994) has recently been published.

Test of Adolescent and Adult Language—3 (Hammill et al., 1994)

Age range: 12;0–24;0. This test assesses verbal comprehension and expression, reading and writing skills and provides normative data from American adolescent populations.

Test of Adolescent/Adult Word Finding (German, 1990)

Age range: 12;0 to adulthood. This test assesses confrontation naming skills at a single word level over a range of tasks. Normative values for speed of response and naming accuracy are given for an American population.

Discourse analysis

Damico (1985) identifies a common difficulty with the use of formal tests with the adolescent population, namely their lack of sensitivity with regard to language use. He has designed a clinical discourse analysis framework (p. 176) and this is summarised below. Difficulties at a discourse level are also discussed in the section on differential diagnosis.

• Quantity
    Failure to provide significant information to the listener.
    Use of non-specific vocabulary.

Informational redundancy.
Need for repetition.
- Quality
  Message inaccuracy.
  Relation.
  Poor topic maintenance.
  Inappropriate response.
  Failure to ask relevant questions.
  Situational inappropriateness.
  Inappropriate speech style.
- Manner
  Linguistic non-fluency.
  Revision.
  Delays before responding.
  Failure to structure discourse.
  Turntaking difficulty.
  Gaze inefficiency.
  Inappropriate intonational contour.

Videotape or audiotape recordings of conversational interactions are analysed and behaviours profiled in order to identify problematic areas.

Discussion with adolescent

One of the advantages of working with older children and adolescents is the insight and description of their own difficulties they can bring to the discussion. In addition to the information gathered as outlined in Chapter 2, the adolescent's perception of past and current academic achievement needs exploring in relation to three areas: strengths, weaknesses and any strategies they currently use. The identification of current strategies is extremely important as it may be the strategies themselves which now form part of the presenting problem.

Differential diagnosis of stuttering and language impairment

This section focuses on the assessment framework advocated in this book and identifies areas where issues regarding the differential diagnosis of stuttering and language impairment are likely to emerge.

Characteristics of stuttering behaviour

Stuttering behaviour is categorised as consisting of the following:

- Whole-word repetition.
- Part-word repetition.
- Prolongation.

- Struggle behaviour.
- Other, e.g. physical concommitants, silent blocks.

However, German (1994) discusses word-finding difficulties in discourse and provides the following summary of word-finding characteristics and gives a number of examples to illustrate these behaviours:

- Word or phrase repetitions, e.g. *'I ran, ran to first base'*
- Word reformulations, e.g. *'They were, he was going'*
- Substitutions, e.g. *'Mary bought money.* (target = tickets)
- Insertions, e.g. *'They are at are aa .. I forgot what that is called.'*
- Empty words, e.g. *'Oh it is that thing-a ma-jig you put on the whatcha ma-call-it.'*
- Time fillers, e.g. *'Um, er, ah He is looking through he um, er, ah binoculars.'*
- Delays (prolonged pauses of 6 seconds or more), e.g. *'He is* (8 seconds) *playing* (6 seconds).*'* (German, 1994, p. 327.)

It is clear that any of the above examples could also be used to exemplify common stuttering behaviours. However, part-word repetitions, prolongations, evident struggle, physical concommitants, changes in breathing pattern, e.g. ingressive airstream, mannerisms and tics are not included as characteristics of word-finding behaviours.

Fluency assessment

Echoic speech

The adolescent is required to repeat words which increase in complexity both in terms of number of syllables and sound combinations. As discussed earlier, some adolescents with language impairment may have residual difficulties with these words and this needs to be borne in mind when analysing results. Careful examination of written work may yield further information in these cases.

Reading aloud (2 minutes)

Any difficulties with this task are analysed with reference to the range of stuttering behaviours outlined above. Word substitutions are of particular interest. These may be indicative of avoidance behaviour relating to dysfluency, for example, substitution of a word with similar meaning in order to avoid a specific initial sound. Alternately, substitution may be an indicator of a reading difficulty. Miscue analysis is a form of reading assessment in which errors made whilst reading aloud are recorded and subsequently analysed. Moon (1990) describes a very basic form of miscue analysis in which any word that is substituted is rated in terms of similarity to the target word on four characteristics:

1. Sound (usually the same initial sound is used).
2. Look (length and shape of word).
3. Part of speech (same word class).
4. Meaning (is meaning retained?).

In addition, a tally of refusals to read words is also kept. Moon (1990) gives several examples of substitutions (Table 7.1).

Table 7.1 Examples of substitutions (Moon, 1990)

Word printed	Word read	Sound	Look	Part of speech	Meaning retained
grew	gave	✔	✔	✔	✗
tiny	small	✗	✗	✔	✔
never	not	✔	✗	✔	✔
let us	let's	✔	✔	✔	✔
soon	sons	✔	✔	✗	✗
money	ticket	✗	✗	✔	✗

The resultant profile helps to identify the type of strategy the reader is using. For example, if most crosses fall in the final column (Meaning retained), with both the sound and look of the word remaining similar, the person is using a phonologically based reading strategy. If meaning is maintained but the substituted word is dissimilar in terms of appearance and initial sound, the reader may be using context (either linguistic or visual) to predict words and may have difficulty in decoding novel words. It is rare for an adolescent to be asked to read aloud as a form of reading skill assessment. However, adolescents with language impairment may have significant difficulties with reading, both at the level of decoding and assimilating meaning. Subtle difficulties in oral reading tasks may be one of the first indications of a possible underlying language impairment.

In terms of differentiating between a stuttering behaviour and a reading–language-related behaviour, one would anticipate that an adolescent who stutters but does not have any other associated difficulties would have a profile in which the initial sound and the appearance of the word might vary considerably from the target word but the meaning and word class would be maintained.

Discourse

Paucity of output and simplistic expression of ideas may be indicative of language difficulties. Difficulty in establishing or maintaining topic, use of redundant information and delay in response may be attributable to word-finding or discourse difficulties or stuttering behaviours. Damico

(1985) gives several examples of difficulties which could be open to several interpretations and illustrates the complexity in trying to identify causation at a discourse level. For example:

* Use of non-specific vocabulary
  Examiner: Well then, what is your favourite toy?
  'My favourite thing is ... oh, stuff.'
* Linguistic non-fluency (the person searches for words and appropriate syntax to code a thought, a temporal mapping problem) 'Sh ... uh ... she ... um ... she comes at dinner.'

Intervention

In an ideal situation the adolescent's language needs should be addressed within the context of the curriculum. There should be liaison between the speech and language therapist and the school-based learning support department. In this way specific language aims can be achieved through adaptation of the curriculum and with the involvement of those working with the adolescent on an ongoing basis. Unfortunately, many therapists will be unable to work in this way due to both time and caseload constraints. However, there are a number of commercially produced intervention packages which provide systematic and graded programmes of work, for example, the *HELP* series (Lazzari and Peters, 1987); the *Word Finding Intervention Program* (German, 1993), and *Question the Information—Techniques for Classroom Listening* (Danielson and Sampson, 1992). These can provide a useful basis for planning a combined clinic and home management programme.

The development of basic compensatory strategies is also achievable within the context of clinic- and home-based work and links strongly with aspects of the fluency work, for example, use of brainstorming and problem-solving.

Discussion with the adolescent regarding the nature of his language difficulties and their impact on communication and learning will help to develop insight into why certain tasks are difficult. This, in turn, will help the adolescent who stutters to view any dysfluency within a realistic frame of reference which contains information about other aspects of social and educational functioning.

Two case studies are now discussed in detail in order to exemplify the points made so far.

Case study

'Hugh was referred at age 15;1. He had a mild to moderate stutter (7%) and had not been seen previously by a speech and language therapist. Hugh's early language development was described as slow, with first words at approximately 15 months and these were very unclear. Hugh's speech remained unclear until he was approximately 5 years old, but intelligibility had improved sufficiently for him to be understood on school entry. He had a period of ear infections at about 2 years old. In addition, there was a family history of literacy difficulties.'

Description of current areas of strength and difficulty

'Hugh's favourite subjects were art, drama, sport and English. He identified his main difficulties as spelling and keeping up with notetaking and dictation. He started off well in written tasks but was unable to maintain the level of output necessary. This resulted in his writing becoming more and more frag-mented, with the loss of both content and structure. Hugh also reported diffi-culty in learning new words, particularly if they were polysyllabic. A recent example had been the word 'Inverness'. Initially, Hugh could remember the first part of the word but it had taken several repetitions before the whole word had been learnt. He had also experienced difficulty in retrieving words. This was particularly noticeable in stressful situations when rapid responses were required, e.g. answering within class. Hugh received private tuition and it had been noted that he could not discriminate between the sounds 'f' and 'th', (as in *thin*) and 'v' and 'th', (as in *the*) even though he was able to use the sounds appropriately and this was affecting his spelling.

Assessment findings

Formal assessment

Receptive and expressive skills were assessed by use of the *British Picture Vocabulary Scales* (BPVS) and the *Clinical Evaluation of Language Funda-mentals—Revised* (CELF-R) and the results were as follows:

BPVS
Raw score: 124
Standard score: 102
Age equivalent: 14;11
Confidence interval: 14;1–15;11

CELF-R
Total language score: 99 (normal range 85–115)
Age equivalent: 15;5

which was made up of the following:

Receptive language score: 112
Expressive language score: 86.

This indicates a discrepancy between receptive and expressive language skills, although both fall within normal limits. This quantitative information was helpful in establishing a baseline skill level. However, it was the qualita-tive aspects of his performance on individual subtests which was indicative of where some of his specific difficulties lay.

On tasks which required a motor response, such as pointing, Hugh responded rapidly and decisively, e.g. oral directions subtest.

Tasks which required the retention of verbal material which then had to be manipulated internally before formulating a response produced a different profile.

Word association

In this subtest four words are presented verbally and the link between two of them has to be identified. Hugh scored 100% but what was so marked was the length of time it took to identify a link. This amounted to several minutes on later items. He had no difficulty in retaining the words in his memory and did not ask for any repetitions.

Formulated sentences

In this subtest one or two key words are given and these then have to be included in a novel sentence. Again, the outstanding feature was the amount of time required by Hugh before formulating a response and this stretched into several minutes for later items. The sentences he generated were syntactically complex, e.g. Given the words 'before' and 'if' he responded with *'It's an hour before my flight goes if I took the boat I wouldn't have to wait so long'.*

Word classes

Given a broad category heading, such as 'animals', the person has to generate as many names as possible in 60 seconds. Although he scored within normal limits Hugh appeared to experience considerable stress during this task as evidenced by his finger drumming and calling himself 'stupid' under his breath as he searched for words.

Assessment of speech discrimination skills

Speech discrimination skills were assessed in several ways:

- Same/different judgements, e.g. pin/pin, mop/mob, mof/nof. Using non-word and real word pairs Hugh was able to discriminate all pairs apart from those contrasting f–th and v–th in initial, medial and final positions.
- Minimal pair discrimination, e.g. pan/fan, four/saw. Hugh's difficulties reflected those experienced in the preceding task, i.e. he was unable to discriminate between pairs involving f, v and th. In addition, he had difficulty discriminating between, fan/van, mouth/mouse, seat/feet, wing/ring, sum/sun, head/hen, grass/glass, train/chain.

On completion of assessment the following recommendations were made in relation to his language needs:

1. A speech discrimination programme. This was carried out at home by Hugh and his mother and monitored by the speech and language therapist. This involved discriminating between pairs of sounds in increasingly complex contexts, i.e. from sounds in isolation to words in short sentences.
2. Inclusion of exercises on word-building skills to be included in his literacy support programme. These focused at the phonological level, e.g. anagrams, segmentation tasks, affix patterns.
3. A short advisory programme to develop self-cuing techniques for word

retrieval. This focused on imagery and semantic links as these were areas of relative strength, e.g. lead in phrases such as 'knife and ...', word length.

4. Strategy development for notetaking, e.g. identifying key information. In addition, Hugh was given information about study skill courses available for young adults with specific language disorder.

5. Development of strategies to increase written output, e.g. use of brainstorming, mind maps and graphic organisers to prepare written work. Use of tape recorder to record initial ideas verbally before writing.

6. The suitability of word processing packages was investigated as some contain grammar checks and predictive spelling packages in addition to conventional spellcheckers.

7. Considerable time was spent in discussion with Hugh so that as he gained insight into both his strengths and areas of difficulty he would begin to understand why certain tasks are particularly problematic. He also needed to learn not to exacerbate his difficulties by placing himself under additional pressure through inaccurate perception of his performance.

8. Hugh attended a social skills course so that he could develop skills in facilitating interactions, e.g. keeping the listener informed when he was experiencing difficulties. This was achieved by use of key phrases such as *'I need time to think'*, *'I'm searching for a particular word'*. Social skills would become increasingly important as he prepared to leave school, attend interviews and encounter unfamiliar people on a regular basis.

9. Hugh's difficulties at a language processing level had been previously undetected, the focus being on his written skills. The recognition that Hugh needed additional time not only to write but also to formulate his ideas was crucial. All possibilities were explored in terms of what types of support were available for written exams, e.g. whether or not a scribe could be used when a high level of written output was required. The school canvassed opinion among teachers about the use of a dictaphone in class in place of taking written notes, and this was agreed.

Case study

'Malcolm, at age 14;6, presented with a moderate to severe stutter (11%). In addition, he had high-level receptive and expressive language difficulties, which manifested as a 2-year delay on formal assessment measures (BPVS, CELF-R). The functional implications of his language impairment within the educational context were identified as follows:

• A generalised difficulty in following complex instructions given to the whole class.
• Difficulty with specific skills, such as prediction and inference, sequencing events, attending to key information and drawing conclusions.

He was receiving individual teaching support for several hours every week and his apparent inability to paraphrase written information had been highlighted as an area of particular concern. Discussion with Malcolm revealed that in primary school he had developed a strategy for matching key words in a written question with the same word in the text and copying out the relevant sentence or paragraph as his answer. He had found this to be a successful strategy in completing work assignments and had continued to use it once he entered secondary school. However, the curriculum demands had changed and there was an expectation that pupils should start to interpret the material in a more sophisticated way, e.g. the use of expository styles of writing. Unfortunately, Malcolm's strategy prevented him from acquiring this skill and the identification and development of new strategies would need to form part of his management programme. Following the initial assessment and with Malcolm's consent, his individual support teacher was contacted by telephone. In addition to the difficulties already identified she expressed concern regarding Malcolm's passive response in whole class situations where he did not understand the requirements of the task.

Management programme

The programme was divided into four parts:

1. Specific skill development. A series of graded reading paragraphs (*Living and Learning*, 1983) were used as the basis to provide structured activities at home. They were used to develop both understanding of written and spoken language.
2. Comprehension monitoring. Malcolm worked on this area both at home and at school with the help of his individual support teacher. At home, Malcolm focused on identifying vocabulary difficulties when working from textbooks. Initially, he read a short section of text aloud to one of his parents. Key vocabulary items were recorded on a chart and an asterisk put beside any word that Malcolm had particular difficulty in reading. Malcolm would rate each word according to how well he felt he knew it. Levels of word knowledge were verified by Malcolm giving a short definition of words he thought he knew well. He then decided on what action to take for unknown words, e.g. look up the meaning in a dictionary, ask the teacher in the next lesson. Finally, he had to record that he had completed the action and rate his word knowledge again and then file the vocabulary sheet so that it was available for future reference at examination time.

Example of Malcolm's identification of vocabulary difficulties

Word	Know well	Know slightly	Don't know	Action	Done
compensatory	✔			None	
liquidation		✔		Ask teacher	14.11.94
fulfilled			✔	Look up in dictionary	19.11.94
strategic			✔	Look up in dictionary	19.11.94

Documenting appropriate action in this way highlighted some interesting findings during the first week. Although Malcolm had access to a range of dictionaries of varying complexity, he rarely suggested this as a way of finding out information. Instead he would advocate discussing the words with his support teacher on her next visit, even if it was several days away. This emphasised how dependant he had become on adults for support and was neglecting to use more immediate strategies.

Once Malcolm was familiar with the task he started to record key vocabulary items himself during silent reading. In the final stage, he only recorded words that were unfamiliar to him.

At school, his main focus was the identification of failure to follow whole class instructions. Rather than automatically repeating or paraphrasing all of the class instructions, his support teacher would now wait until Malcolm requested help. In individual sessions they discussed what Malcolm could do if did not understand an instruction. Each week Malcolm would bring an example of a difficulty he had experienced. He would identify as many different solutions as possible, i.e. brainstorming, and then describe which would be the most appropriate in that particular situation. Having identified a range of strategies Malcolm would select one to try out during the coming week and report back at the next session. Gradually his repertoire of strategies increased and, because of their effectiveness, he began to use them spontaneously in class.

3. Developing a range of written styles of language. In order to support the work aimed at directly improving Malcolm's comprehension of spoken and written text, he was introduced to graphic organisers (Smith and Tompkins, 1988) for a number of common text structures. For example:

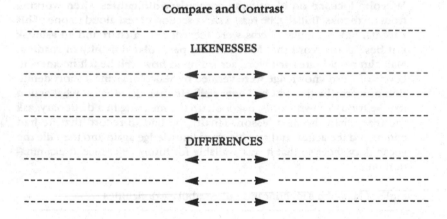

Homework assignments were used, firstly, to identify the type of response required and, secondly, to organise the response within the appropriate framework.

4. Decreasing the external demands by use of teacher-based strategies. Finally, an important element to the total management plan was the inclusion of appropriate teacher-based strategies which maximised Malcolm's functioning within this context. The strategies needed to be simple, easy to incorporate into the existing lesson plan and minimal in terms of time investment for the teacher concerned.

Below are some examples of strategies suggested to support Malcolm. These were discussed by the individual support teacher with subject teachers in the school.

- **Use of visual aids**
  Use of diagrams, written overhead transparencies and slides to support the understanding of spoken language. Pointing out the appropriate part of text or covering over irrelevant material to provide the necessary focus.
- **Presenting new information**
  Use of short sentences and pausing regularly to give Malcolm the opportunity to process the information.
- **Orientation at beginning of the lesson**
  The use of an advance organiser at the beginning of a lesson. A brief resume of the lesson format is given with explicit guidance as to the task demands.

Example
'Today we are starting a new topic which is 'Artificial Intelligence'. (PAUSE)
'I am going to talk to you for about 15 minutes and then you will do some group work.' (PAUSE)
'You will need to make notes on what I am saying because there will be a short test in 2 weeks' time.' (PAUSE)
'Any questions?' (PAUSE)
'Are you ready to start?'
(Looks at whole class and makes sure Malcolm gives visual sign of understanding and readiness, e.g. head nod)
'Good...'

Summary

In this chapter we have explored the potential relationship between stuttering and language impairment. We have discussed a particular model of language processing and how the adoption of this model affects both assessment and intervention. Issues relating to assessment, differential diagnosis and intervention have been identified and exemplified by two case studies. A number of sources of further reading have been identified.

The positive link between stuttering and language impairment has yet to be confirmed. However, given our understanding of the nature of language impairment and its manifestations in adolescence, it is clear that the assessment of language skills needs to form an integral part of the fluency assessment. Any identified needs may then be addressed within the total management plan.

Appendices

Appendix I Fluency assessment

Initial Assessment Form

2

Summary of Results *(Time should be converted to minutes, using round-up rules below*)*

| Total stuttered words (SW) | | = | stuttered words per minute (SW/M) | | | Total stuttered words (SW) | | | Total words spoken (WS) | | | = | words spoken per minute (WS/M) | | |
| Total time (minutes) | | | | | | Total words spoken (WS) | | | Total time (minutes) | | | | | | |

Type of Stutter *(Tick as applicable)*   whole word repetition (W/w)   prolongation (P)   other behaviour:

part word repetition (P/W) $\dfrac{100}{1} \times \dfrac{}{}$ = ___ % stuttered words   struggle behaviour (S)

Task	Automatic Speech	Echoic Speech	Reading (Optional)	Naming	Monologue	Questions	Conversation	Remarks
	Ask the child to: count to 20 name the days of the week recite a nursery rhyme	Say after me, one at a time, these words: tea men at hello coffee present enormous institution establishment occupational categorically come home the horse under the chair I want a biscuit it's a funny thing tomorrow we are going to the park	Ask the child to read aloud for two minutes	Ask the child to name 10 pictures	Talk to me about anything you like for two minutes (School, hobbies, holidays, pets, home, etc.)	What is your name? Where do you go to school/work? How do you get there? How many are there in your family? What can you tell me about them? Now you ask me five questions	Engage the child in conversation for two minutes	
Time (Seconds)								**Total Time (Secs)**
Stuttered Words								**Total Stuttered Words**
Words Spoken								**Total Words Spoken**

		Total Time (Mins)

*Round-up rules for time: 7 to 22 secs = 0.25 min; 23 to 36 secs = 0.50 min; 37 to 52 secs = 0.75 min: 53 secs to 1 min. 6 secs = 1.0 min

Reproduced with kind permission of NFER-NELSON.

Appendix II Adolescent interview

NAME: DOB:

HOME ADDRESS:

TEL:

SCHOOL:
(including address and telephone)

GP:
(including address and telephone)

DATE OF INTERVIEW:
DATE OF REFERRAL:
INTERVIEWER:
NAME OF MOTHER:
NAME OF FATHER:
REFERRING THERAPIST:
(including address and telephone)

First language: Language spoken at home:

NOTES:

SECTION A: SPEECH
Present complaint:
What is the problem as you see it?
Why do you think you have come here today?
Do you have any other problems?
If yes, which one concerns you most?

Detailed description of stuttering:
Describe what happens when you stutter?
(repetition of whole words/part words, whole sentences or phrases?
prolongation, struggle, blocking, avoidance of words, other?)
When did the problem first start? Suddenly or gradually?
Any major events at that time?
Any long periods of fluency?
What do you think caused the stammer?

Frequency:
How often does the problem occur now?

Severity:
How do you rate the severity of the problem on a scale of 1–9?
(1 = extremely mild; 9 = severe)
1 —— 2 —— 3 —— 4 —— 5 —— 6 —— 7 —— 8 —— 9
Are there any other people who stutter in your family?

Self-help strategies:
How do you help yourself become more fluent?
How is that helpful?
How often does it work for you?

☐ Rarely   ☐ Sometimes   ☐ Always

Did you work this out for yourself?

Reactions to stuttering:
Do you know any other stutterers?
How do people react when you stutter?
Mother?
Father?
Siblings?
Friends?
Teachers?
How do you feel about these reactions?
How would you like people to react when you stutter?
How do you feel when you stutter?
How do you think your stutter affects your family?
Whose decision was it to refer you here?

General health:
How is your general health? Do you miss much school through sickness?
Have you been to any other clinic/hospital for any reason, e.g. sight/hear-
ing/psychological?
Ever been an inpatient?
Outpatient?
Any medication or physical problems? Asthma? Eczema?
Are you right- or left-handed?
Right or left footed?
Right or left eyed?

SECTION B: SCHOOL
Type of school:
Single sex or mixed? Boarding or day school? Comprehensive, grammar,

private or other?
What do you think of your school?
Tell me about the discipline in your school
What do you think about the teachers?
Good teachers? (name one)
What makes him/her a good teacher?
Problem teachers (name one)
What's the problem?
What subjects are you currently studying?
To what level?
Favourite subject?
Why?
Least favourite subject?
Why?
Do you have any reading or spelling difficulties?
Difficulties with any other subjects?
How much homework do you receive from school on average?
Any problems?
Are you in the top or bottom half of your class?
Do your parents have regular contact with your school? How often on average?

Exams/qualifications:
Have you recently taken any exams?
Passes? Fails?
Any exams in the near future?
How do you feel about taking exams?
Any studying difficulties?

Career plans:
What plans do you have on leaving school?
Can you foresee any problems in achieving your career goals?

Sex education:
Have you been instructed in sexual matters?
Are you satisfied with the information you've received?
If you wanted further information where would you go?
(Girls) Have you started menstruation? Age? Any problems?
Are you interested in the opposite sex?
Do you have a girlfriend/boyfriend?
Name? Age?
If yes; how long have you been going out with each other?
What's he/she like?
How do you get on with each other?
If no; Have you ever had a boyfriend/girlfriend?

Would you like a boyfriend/girlfriend?

Peer relationships:
Do you have any friends at school? Do you see them outside of school?
Names:
Do you have other friends outside school?
Names:
Are they mostly boys or girls or a mixture?
Are they the same age as you? Older? Younger?

Social life:
How do you spend your evenings and weekends?
What do you like doing with your friends?
What interests and hobbies do you have?
Are you a member of any clubs or organisations?
What's your favourite type of music?
What's your favourite food?
Do you have any eating problems?
Do you have a part time job?
Do you get any pocket money?
How much?
What do you spend your money on?

Bullying/teasing:
Do you ever get picked on or teased or bullied?
By whom?
Describe it (Verbal? Physical?)
What's it about usually?
If a problem, how do you manage it?
Do you bully or tease others?
Have you ever truanted or refused to go to school? Why?

SECTION C: HOME
Do you live in a house or flat?
Do you have your own room? Sleeping arrangements in home?
Number of bedrooms?
Do you help out in the home? What tasks or jobs do you do?

Siblings:
Do you have any brothers or sisters?
Names?
Ages?
Position in family?
Are they all living at home?
(if not describe circumstances)

Do any of them have any problems?
How do you get on with them?
Do you ever argue or fight?
With whom?
Who are you closest to you? Why?

Parents:
What is your parents religion and what religion are you?
What languages are spoken at home/what is your first language?
Mother and Father both living at home?
How do your parents get on with each other?
How do you get on with:
Mother?
Father?
Which one do you relate to more easily?
Why?
In what ways do your parents get on your nerves?
Who do you think is your mother's favourite in your family?
Father's favourite?
In what ways do you get on your parents nerves?
Do you go out as a family? How often?
Do you think there are any problems in your family?
Are there any other adults/older people you get on well with?

Discipline in the home:
Who does most of the reprimanding in your home?
How are you punished?
What time do you go to bed?
Weekdays: Weekends:
What time do you get up in the mornings?
Are you allowed to leave the house without saying where you are going?
Are there any restrictions on: friends? reading materials? television watched?
videos watched?
Do you have your own television?
Video games?
Have you ever been in trouble with the police?
Ever been to court?
Do you smoke?
How many?
Do you drink?
How much on average in a week?
Any history of alcoholism in your family?
Have you ever been offered any drugs/solvents? By whom?
Have you tried drugs/solvents?

Yes: Which ones?
Are you a regular user?
How do you get hold of them?
How do you pay for them?

SECTION D: CONCEPTS
What's the best thing that's ever happened to you?
What's the worst thing?
Tell me three good things and three not such good things about you?
Are you a leader or a follower?
Do you worry?
What about?
Do you have a temper?
How is this shown?
Do you have any fears or phobias?
What do you do if you have a problem?
How do you react if things go wrong for you?
How do you react if you see a person or an animal hurt?
If there was one thing in your life you could change, what would it be?

SECTION E: SPEECH THERAPY
Have you had speech therapy before?
Dates? Duration? Frequency? Type of Activity/Therapy?
Has it been helpful?
If yes, what would you say has helped you?
If not, why do you think this is?
What are you expecting to gain now from speech therapy?
How would life be different if you didn't stutter?
If you had one wish, what would it be?

Separations:
Have you ever stayed away from home without your parents?
How did you get on?
Do you think there is anything else we need to know?
Are there any questions you would like to ask me?

SECTION F: DESCRIPTION OF CLIENT AND REACTION TO INTERVIEW
1) Overall appearance/presentation
   Size?
   Maturity?
2) Anxiety?
3) Tension?
4) Spontaneity of talk/rapport
5) Emotional expressiveness

6) Evidence of avoidance
7) Habitual mannerisms/concomitant behaviours
8) Observation skills?
9) Listening skills
10) Turntaking skills
11) Reinforcement/confidence
12) Problem-solving

SECTION G: MODIFICATION OF STUTTERING BEHAVIOUR
Therapist reduces rate:
Instructs subject to say word fluently
One-word utterances

Therapist models:
Slow rate
Easy onset
Soft contacts
Smooth speech

Recommended technique:

SUMMARY OF ISSUES

FUTURE MANAGEMENT

Appendix III Facts about stuttering

Current research indicates that stuttering is the result of a number of co-existing factors including physical, linguistic, psychological and environmental.

1. The predisposition to stutter is inherited, therefore it may run in families.
2. Stuttering is, in the main, a disorder of childhood with its onset usually between 2 and 5 years.
3. More males than females stutter.
4. Many people who stutter are slightly less skillful with their speech motor processing; therefore the faster they try to talk, the more likely they are to stutter. This means that often more time is needed to coordinate the speech muscles, therefore slowing down can help.
5. Stuttering is reported in all cultures and in all social groups. It has been recorded throughout history.
6. The longer that a person has been stuttering, the less chance he or she has of 'growing out of it'.
7. Although no differences in personality factors have been found, people who stutter may develop some difficulties in social relationships.
8. Parents do not 'cause' stuttering, but can influence progress.

Appendix IV Assessment booklet

 ASSESSMENT AND THERAPY
PROGRAMME FOR DYSFLUENT CHILDREN
Lena Rustin

Assessment Booklet

Child

Family name: ....

First name(s): ....

Sex: .... Date of birth: .... Age on date of interview: ....

School: ....

Home address: ....

....

.... Tel: ....

Parents

Mother   ### Father

Family name: ....   Family name: ....

First name(s): ....   First name(s): ....

Address, if different from child's address: ....

....

....

.... Tel: ....

Interviewer: ....Date: ....

The NFER-NELSON Publishing Company Ltd., a joint venture of the
National Foundation for Educational Research in England and Wales
and Thomas Nelson and Sons Ltd., Educational Publishers.

© Lena Rustin, 1987

All rights reserved. No part of this publication may be reproduced, stored in a retrieval system,
or transmitted in any form or by any means, electronic, mechanical, photocopying, recording,
or otherwise, even within the terms of a Photocopying Licence, without the prior permission of
the publishers.
Published by The NFER-NELSON Publishing Company Ltd.,
Darville House, 2 Oxford Road East, Windsor, Berkshire SL1 1DF (0753-858961)
Code: 4044 03 4 (Client Pack) 1(11.87)
Note: the Child Assessment is a separate section, enclosed in the centre of this Booklet.

Parental Interview

Present Complaint

Detailed description of stuttering

How is the behaviour shown?

Date of onset?

Any major events at this time?

Frequency?   Severity?

Context: When is the stutter worst?

When is the stutter least?

What do you do when your child stutters?

Mother:

Father:

Other members of family:

How does the stutter affect the family?

Why are you seeking help now?

Recent behaviour and emotional state

General health

Away from school?   Stomach aches?

Asthma?   Sight?

Headaches?   Hearing?

Eating, sleeping and elimination

Eating difficulties at home or school?

Sleeping difficulties?

Nightmares?   Talking in sleep?

Sleepwalking?   Enuresis?   Soiling?

Regular bowel movement?

Muscular system and concentration

Overactive or restless?   Stay still if expected to?   Fidgety?

Concentration?   Longest time on something interesting?

Clumsiness?   Preferred hand and foot?

Speech

Speak as well as others of same age?   Difficulties in pronunciation?

Spontaneity of talking?

Tics and mannerisms

Twitches face or shoulders?   Nail-biting?

Blinking?   Headbanging?

Sucking thumb?   Soft toy or blanket?

Attack disorders

Faints?   Fits?   Petit Mal?

Emotions

Happy or miserable?   Crying?
Worried?

Irritable?

Temper?   Fears?   Sulking?
Tears on going to school?   School refusal?
Fussy?   Rituals?

Peer relationships

How does the child get on with other children?
Friends?   See them outside school?
Prefers children of own age?   Younger or older?
Girls or boys?   Leader or follower?
Bully?   Bullied?   Fights?
Teased?   Member of club?

Relationship with siblings

Position in the family?
Names and ages of siblings:
How do they get on?   How is this shown?
Particularly attached to any sibling?
Squabbling?   Who with?
Come to blows?   Jealousy?
Do the siblings have any particular problems?

Relationship with adults

How does the child get on with:
  mother?
  father?
Which child in the family do you relate to more easily?
  mother's reply:
  father's reply:
How does the child compare with other children?
How is affection shown?
Is the child easy to get on with?   Who does the child take after?
In what ways does the child get on your nerves?
  mother's reply:
  father's reply:
How does the child get on with other adults?   With teachers?

Anti-social trends

Disobedient?

Fire setting?

Stealing?

   At home or outside?

Truanting?

Smoke?

Drugs?

Destructive?

Lies?

On own or with others?

Run away?

Drinks?

Trouble with police?

Sex education

Interest in opposite sex?

Instructed in sex?

Masturbation?

Questions asked?

Menstruation?

Schooling

Which school/s attended (including nursery placement)?

Like it?

Progress: Reading?

        Writing?

        Other?

Reports?

Do parents see the teacher?

Family structure and history

How long married/together?

Previous marriages/children?

Previous long-term relationships/children?

Mother's pregnancies, abortions, miscarriages or still births?

Children adopted or fostered?

Number in home?

Personal background	Mother	Father
Place of birth		
Age		
Religion		
Occupation		
Education		
General health/illness		

Personal background	Mother	Father
Description of personality		
Depression?		
Seen by psychiatrist?		
Difficulty learning to read or speak		
Emotional problems		
Stuttering (any treatment?)		
Left-handed		
Enuretic		
Alcoholism		
Epilepsy		
Court appearances		

Parents' family background	Mother	Father
Siblings		
Upbringing		

The child's grandparents	Maternal grandparents	Paternal grandparents
Occupation		
Current contact		
(Date and cause of death)		

Extended family issues	Mother's family	Father's family
Psychiatric treatment		
Depression		
Suicide/attempt		
Slow to speak		
Stuttering		
Difficulty learning to read		
Left handed		
Enuretic		
Mental illness		
Alcoholism		
Epilepsy		
Court appearances		

Home circumstances

House or flat?   Number of bedrooms?

Sleeping arrangements?   Others in home?

Finances

Any difficulties?

Neighbourhood

How long lived there?   Do you like it?

Family life and relationships

Parental relationships

How do you get on?

Things enjoyed doing together?

How spend evenings and weekends?

Father's participation in child care and household tasks?

How would the child's life be different is he did not stutter?

How do parents resolve problems in the family?

Parent-child interaction

Activities child enjoys?

Go out together?

Play together?

Help with homework?   Help make things?

Child's participation in family activities

Help with dressing?   Feeding?   Who helps?

Taken to school?

Does the child help with washing up, shopping, errands, etc?

Family relationships

Is the child a 'mother's child' or a 'father's child'?

Confide in father?

       mother?

Attachment to other adults?

Discipline

Bedtime regulations (including time?)

Allowed to climb on furniture?   Allowed to leave house without saying where going?

Restrictions on friends: Reading: TV:

Who reprimands?

What method of punishment is used?

Pocket money?   Amount:

Child's developmental history

Pregnancy

Mother's health during pregnancy?

Home or hospital delivery?

Maturity?   Birthweight?

Health after pregnancy?

Neonatal period

Difficulties breathing or sucking?

Convulsions?   Jaundice?

Feeding

Breast or bottle?   Weaning when?   Introduction of solids?

Development in infancy

Placid or active?   Crying?   Response to mother?

Milestones

Sitting unsupported?   Walking?

First words with meaning?   First three-word phrases?

Comparison with siblings?

Any developmental problems?

Bladder and bowel control

When obtained?

Day: . Night: Problems:

Illnesses

Ever been in hospital? In patient:

                         Outpatient:

Clinic: (a) Speech

        (b) Child guidance

        (c) Other, including accident and emergency

Serious illnesses?

Separations

Ever away from home without parents?

Apart from parents (holidays, hospitals, etc)

How looked after?

Reaction?

Other comments

Temperamental or personality attributes

Meeting new people

Adults?   Children?

Go up to strangers?

Shy or clinging?   How quickly does the child adapt to someone new?

New situations

Reaction to: (a) New places: does the child explore or hang back?

             (b) New gadgets?

             (c) New foods?

How quick to adapt?

Emotional expression

How vigorous in expression of feelings?

Sensitivity

How does the child respond if a person or an animal is hurt?

How does the child react if something goes wrong?

Additional comments

Note rate of parents' speech

Note future impending changes

How do parents resolve problems in the family?

Summary of issues

Management

Appendix V Checklist of social skills

To be completed on day (1)

Name: Date:

1) Eye-contact (when speaking and listening).

2) Facial expression (when speaking and listening).

3) Body posture.

4) Observation skills.

5) Attention and listening skills.

6) Verbal skills (e.g. content of speech).

7) Volume/pitch/intonation/rate.

8) Meshing skills (e.g. flow, timing, turntaking).

9) Social routines:
    Greetings/parting.
    Requests.
    Approaching strangers.
    Remedial routines.
    Assertion.

10) Negotiation skills.

11) Other comments.

Appendix VI Social communication skills Self-rating scale

Name: Date:

Please rate your skills in the following areas:	never good	rarely good	sometimes good	often good	always good
1) Looking at people when I'm talking to them and they are talking to me					
2) Listening to what other people have to say					
3) Starting a conversation					
4) Taking turns in a conversation					
5) Asking questions					
6) Answering questions					
7) Maintaining an appropriate distance between myself and others when I'm talking					
8) Praising other people					
9) Disagreeing with others					
10) Agreeing with others					
11) Finding solutions to problems					
12) Talking at the right speed (not too fast, not too slow)					

TOTAL   %

Appendix VII Measurement of change and outcome

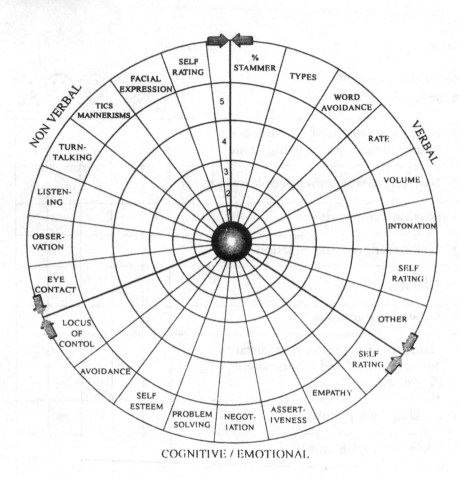

Appendix VIII Measurements of change

CATEGORY ONE: Verbal

Stutter:
    1. > 20%
    2. < 20%
    3. < 15%
    4. < 10%
    5. < 3%

Types:
    1. repetitions, prolongations, struggle, concomitants
    2. repetitions, struggle, blocking
    3. repetitions, prolongations
    4. repetitions (part-word and whole word)
    5. normal non-fluencies

Avoidances (verbal):
    1. persistent, majority of speaking situations.
    2. frequent, daily, many situations
    3. often, most days, predictable in certain situations
    4. sometimes, certain situations
    5. always attempts word, never tries to avoid

Speech rate:
    1. > 150 wpm
    2. 140–150 wpm
    3. 130–140 wpm
    4. 120–130 wpm
    5. controlled and appropriate

Volume:
    1. extreme, inappropriate
    2. frequently a problem
    3. often a problem
    4. occasionally a problem
    5. appropriate use

Intonation:
    1. monotonous
    2. frequently monotonous
    3. occasionally good
    4. often good
    5. normal

Self-rating:
    1. severe, persistent problem
    2. frequently a problem
    3. often a problem
    4. occasionally a problem
    5. seldom a problem

CATEGORY TWO: Non-verbal

Eye-contact:

1. very poor
2. limited, frequently avoided
3. appropriate in some situations
4. minimal problem
5. normal—speaker and listener

Observation:

1. subjective, self centred perceptions, all situations
2. judgements focused around stuttering
3. evaluations of some situations realistic
4. often objective/realistic
5. observations realistic, accurate

Listening:

1. distracted, appears not listen
2. poor listening, often distracted
3. sometimes giving signs of listening
4. often listens appropriate, offers evidence
5. appropriate

Turntaking:

1. inappropriate interruptions, holds turn
2. noticeable difficulty
3. sometimes able to take or offer turn
4. often able to participate equally
5. appropriate

Mannerisms/tics:

1. constant concomitants and mannerisms
2. frequent extraneous movements
3. some extraneous movements
4. occasional extraneous movements
5. appropriate, non-distracting

Facial expression:

1. usually inappropriate
2. frequently inappropriate
3. sometimes inappropriate
5. appropriate to situation

Self-rating:

1. usually a problem
2. frequently a problem
3. sometimes a problem
4. usually good
5. always appropriate.

CATEGORY THREE: Cognitive–emotional

Locus of control:
1. strongly external
2. external, particularly regarding stuttering
3. aware of aspects of self determination
4. clear evidence of self determination
5. internalised

Situational avoidance:
1. usually avoids stressful speaking situations
2. frequently avoids
3. often
4. sometimes
5. attempts all situations

Self-esteem:
1. low, feelings of inadequacy, failure
2. frequently feels lack of confidence
3. aware of certain skills, and some confidence
4. often confident in certain situations
5. adequate levels of self-esteem

Problem-solving:
1. no strategies, expectations of others/chance
2. often feel helpless
3. some strategies in certain areas
4. useful strategies, often used
5. good problem solving, 'owns' problem

Negotiation:
1. no ability
2. some attempts
3. attempts and identifies alternatives
4. frequent use of strategies
5. good negotiation skills, understand strategies

Assertiveness:
1. aggressive/passive
2. occasional attempts
3. sometimes successful
4. ability to assert in many situations
5. assertiveness understood and practical

Empathy:
1. little understanding of others' perceptions
2. some understanding
3. readiness to understand others perceptions
4. frequent attempts at empathizing
5. empathic

Self-rating:

1. severe problem, no control
2. moderate problem, occasional control
3. some control in certain circumstances
4. usually in control
5. taking responsibility, understands variations.

These ratings are, in the main, subjective, although some of the objective measurements contribute to scoring. It would be recommended that speech and language therapists define their own scoring in detail when working alone for re-test reliability, or that team members discuss each section fully to gain inter-rater reliability in scoring.

This system for measuring progress and outcomes is part of an ongoing study.

Appendix IX The communication skills course Intensive group therapy course workbook

WELCOME TO TWO WEEKS OF HARD WORK, DEMANDING ACTIVITIES AND ... ENJOYMENT!

THIS IS YOUR WORKBOOK. IT IS INTENDED AS YOUR OWN PERSONAL RECORD OF THE WORK YOU WILL BE DOING ON THE COURSE, YOUR ACHIEVEMENTS AND PROGRESS. PLEASE ENSURE THAT YOU KEEP IT SAFE AND SECURE AND THAT YOU UPDATE IT AT REGULAR INTERVALS. WE ENCOURAGE YOU TO WRITE DOWN ANY THOUGHTS AND IDEAS WHICH MAY OCCUR TO YOU DURING THIS TWO WEEKS EXPERIENCE—SOME OF WHICH YOU MAY WISH TO DISCUSS WITH STAFF OR OTHER GROUP MEMBERS, SOME OF WHICH YOU MAY WISH TO KEEP TO YOURSELF—THAT'S YOUR CHOICE.

About the course:

This intensive course has been evolving over the past 20 years. We are therefore confident that we are offering the best therapy available. Every group differs because of the individuality of each, we do try to adapt exercises and activities for the needs of the group.

The programme is called THE COMMUNICATION SKILLS APPROACH. As you go through the course with us, you will gain a complete understanding of why we talk about communications rather than fluency.

There is a daily schedule of targets, with activities and exercises designed to develop all aspects of communication. Opportunity for discussion is given following each exercise and at the end of the day. Feedback is welcomed.

Parents attend on one day of the course. They form a separate group which gives them the chance to gain a better understanding of what we are aiming to achieve and possible ways in which they can be helpful.

The first day of the course is quite different from the rest. It is a priority that we all get to know each other so that we can work well together. Activities form the basis for this. In addition there are a number of assessments that we need to complete in order for us to be able to measure progress both during the course and afterwards. The rest of the course is devoted to communication skills.

Please let us know, at any stage, at any time, if you are experiencing problems on the course. AT THE END OF THE DAY, YOU'LL GET AS MUCH OUT OF THE COURSE AS YOU ARE PREPARED TO PUT IN!

EXPECTATIONS OF THE COURSE

COMMUNICATION

SPEECH PRODUCTION

WHAT CAN GO WRONG WITH SPEECH

STUTTERING/STAMMERING

MY STUTTER

WHAT IS FLUENCY?

SPEECH MODIFICATION TECHNIQUE

ACTIONS FOR PROBLEMS:

(reproduced in reduced format)

PRACTISING FLUENCY

MODELLING

Step A is : Therapist only; Therapist and child together; Child only

Step B is : Child only

1A Single Words

1B Single Words

2A Two word Phrases

2B Two Word Phrases

3A Three Word Phrases

3B Three Word Phrases

4A Four Word Phrases

4B Four Word Phrases

5 One sentence

6 Two sentences

7 Three Sentences

8 Timed Speech 30 seconds

9 Modelling Stage Complete

Ref: STAMPRO 5.1

Fluency Stages

Stage One: Reading

1 One word

2 Two words at a time

3 Three words at a time

4 Four words at a time

5 Five words at a time

6 One sentence

Two sentences at a time

Three sentences at a time

Four sentences at a time

Five sentences at a time

7 Timed reading: 30 seconds

1 minute

1½ minutes

2 minutes

Stage One Complete

Stage Two: Picture Description or Monologue

1 Say one word

2 Say two words at a time

3 Say three words at a time

4 Say four words at a time

5 Say five words at a time

6 Say one sentence

   Say two sentences at a time

   Say three sentences at a time

   Say four sentences at a time

   Say five sentences at a time

7 Timed speech: 30 seconds

                    1 minute

                    1½ minutes

                    2 minutes

                                            Stage Two Complete

Stage Three: Conversation

1 Say one word

2 Say two words at a time

3 Say three words at a time

4 Say four words at a time

5 Say five words at a time

6 Say one sentence

   Say two sentences at a time

   Say three sentences at a time

   Say four sentences at a time

   Say five sentences at a time

7 Timed speech: 30 seconds

                  1 minute

                  1½ minutes

                  2 minutes

Stage Three Complete

Homework sheet

	Name		*Date*
	Task		*Outcome*

MONDAY

TUESDAY

WEDNESDAY

THURSDAY

FRIDAY

SATURDAY

SUNDAY

Appendix X

Example of self-characterisation

Write a character sketch of yourself as if you were a close friend of yours, someone who knows you very well, probably better than anyone really does, a sympathetic friend.

> 'George is a generally friendly person who enjoys smoking marijuana and is mainly out to have fun and get stoned. He doesn't like liers and can normally tell when a person is being untruthful even though he might not let on. He has a girlfriend called Helen who he has been with on and off for a year on Saturday. He has a job and that is how he pays for ganja and parties. His parents generally buy him clothes. He enjoys life and would like to stay 16 and he's going to skin up in this room.'

Example of self-characterisation

Write a character sketch of yourself as if you were a close friend of yours, someone who knows you very well, probably better than anyone really does, a sympathetic friend.

> 'Jason is a very sensitive person who cares a lot about how he feels about himself and how other people feel about him, although the two are linked. He likes to be sociable and feels most secure with himself when he's got on well with people, but also is comfortable not on his own as well. I suppose you could say he has quite a few friends but he always strives (as much as he can!) to get more, even though he (sometimes) finds it hard to talk to unknown people (especially girls).
>
> He could be described as being reliable, caring and trustworthy, but not, perhaps, to his family to whom he feels isolated and not on the best of terms with. He scrounges far too many things off friends (lifts, money and fags, beer, etc, etc, etc, etc.) and they often get pissed off with him but I don't blame them, but at heart he is generous and when he has money, splashes out appallingly.'

Appendix XI Examples of brainstorm exercises

Examples of 'brainstorms'

WHAT CAN GO WRONG WITH SPEECH?

VOICE PROBLEMS – CANCER OF THE LARYNX – LISP – CAN'T PRONOUNCE SOME SOUNDS – MONOTONOUS – LANGUAGE BARRIERS – DEAFNESS – BLINDNESS – SORE THROAT – BRAIN DAMAGE – CEREBRAL PALSY – DRUNKENNESS – STAMMERING

WHAT IS STUTTERING?

CAN'T SPEAK – SOUNDS GET MIXED UP – LACK OF CONFIDENCE – BRAIN WORKS TOO FAST – LACK OF COORDINATION IN SPEECH MUSCLES – GETTING STUCK – CAUGHT UP – TENSION – TONGUE GETS TONGUE – CAN'T MOVE IT AS FAST AS BRAIN SAYS – VICIOUS CIRCLE OF 'THINK YOU WILL STUTTER, DO STUTTER, STUTTER NEXT TIME' – REPEATING – TIGHT MUSCLES – FRUSTRATION – PEOPLE THINK YOU ARE DAFT – PEOPLE LAUGH – EMBARRASSED – AVOID – USE TRICKS – EFFORT – PUSHING – CAN'T STOP AND START AGAIN – LOOSE BREATH – PUSHING – NOT ENOUGH AIR, RUN OUT – MUCKS UP CONVERSATIONS – TENSION IN STOMACH – LONGER SOUNDS – STUPID

WHAT IS FLUENCY?

EXPRESS YOURSELF – CAN SAY EVERYTHING CLEARLY – SAY WHAT YOU INTENDED – SPEAK WITHOUT STOPS OR INTERRUPTIONS – BETTER EYE-CONTACT – CAN SAY WHAT YOU WANT TO SAY – DON'T HAVE TO SPEAK TOO FAST – SAY ABSOLUTELY ANYTHING – SPEECH FLOWS, NO STOPS, NO PAUSES, NO REPETITIONS, NO MISTAKES – LOADS OF SELF-CONFIDENCE – CAN SPEAK TO ANYONE – CAN TALK IN FRONT OF GROUPS – NEVER AVOID

Appendix XII Communication skills approach

Example of 'brainstorms'

Communication

'thinking'	'interaction'
'phone'	'talking'
'expressing yourself'	'media'
'conversation'	'writing'
'sign language'	'smoke signals'
	'making friends'
'listening'	'understanding'
'looking—eye-contact'	'posture'
'facial expression'	'tone of speech—voice'
'two—way process'	'body language'

Observation. Why is observation important?

'Can observe gesture, facial expressions'
'Need to look at people, so they know you are talking to them'
'Not seem bored'
'Messages less clear if you don't observe person'
'Need to look to see if someone is listening to you'
'So that you can understand properly, helps you listen'
'So that you know when and how to respond'
'To see that you have made sense'
'To see whether people agree'

Listening. Why is listening important to communication?

'Reinforce speaker'
'Know what the conversation is about and what to say next'
'So you know people are interested in what they're saying'
'Shows respect'
'If people don't listen, you have to repeat – boring'
'Conversation will break down if you don't listen'
'If someone doesn't listen, you lose respect for them – get angry'
'If someone doesn't listen, you don't feel like talking to them again'

Praise and reinforcement

'Makes you feel better shows you are interested'
'Makes a favourable impression brings you closer'
'Helps to break the ice'
'Puts the person at ease—good start to friendship'
'Gives the person confidence'
'Makes the conversation more interesting and the other person more 'interested'
'Helps when talking to opposite sex—unless they reject it'

IMPORTANT CHARACTERISTICS

'It's got to be HONEST you must MEAN IT'
'Mustn't PUT PEOPLE DOWN'
'Should be RELEVANT AND APPROPRIATE'

Appendix XIII   Fear of stuttering and ring of confidence

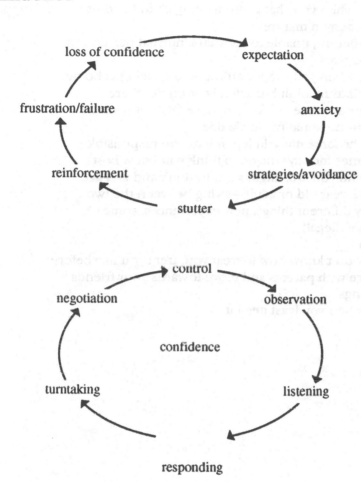

Appendix XIV Adolescents view of adolescence

part of life when you change from being child to adult
   when a person matures
change, different, unable to do what a normal person can
   teenage years
part of life when you change attitudes, e.g. being at home
   feeling like an adult but actually not quite there
most important time of life—you have GCSE's (Exams)
   and your personality can change
when you become more independent and responsible
   sometimes moody—begin to think you know best
not sure who you are, might want to think and and act
   like a 12-year-old or adult—swing between the two
want to try different things, new experiences, some of
   them are illegal!
confusion
   family don't know how to treat you, treat you like before
argue more with parents and move towards your friends
mood swings
pressure when you least need it

Appendix XV How adolescents think parents' view adolescence

    feel rejected
    saddened
kids are angry at home, go out and cause trouble
police stop you because they expect you to cause trouble
    it has happened to them, but they have no experience of looking after
an adolescent if you are their oldest child they've forgotten what its like
    should be seen and not heard
think you've stopped loving them, now hating them
    just doing it to upset them (sometimes true)
they think you are against them all the time, do exact opposite of what
they say
    conflict – they want to prove their own authority
    think you can't accept responsibility, think of you as a child

Appendix XVI Parents' view of adolescence

lazy
money-minded
know it all
moody
selfish
not family-minded
acne
physical changes
oversexed
think they know it all
argumentative
contrary
irresponsible
always right (they think)
angry with parents
rebellious
unapproachable
volatile

Appendix XVII Family session

NAME: DATE:

PRESENT:

1. WHAT DO YOU FEEL _____ HAS GAINED FROM THE COURSE?

A) MOTHER:

B) FATHER:

C) SIBLINGS:

D) CLIENT:

2. (To client) What do you feel you need to do from now on to maintain the gains you have achieved (including follow-up therapy, home practice, etc.)?

3. Do you wish any members of your family to be involved in this plan? Which?

4. (having identified which family members the client is willing to involve) Would you be prepared to help ....? (to each family member identified).

5. How do you want .... to respond to:

a) your fluency?

b) your fluency using speech control?

c) your stuttering?

d) could .... be involved in any aspect of practice?

(Following clarification, each family member is asked whether they agree to the ideas, then—following any necessary negotiation ascertaining feasibility, practicality, etc.—the agreements are carefully written down, for each family member in turn. Each will receive a copy, which is signed by the family member, the client and the therapist.) (Note: this document is reproduced in a reduced format.)

Appendix XVIII Communication skills course

A review

This course has aimed to cover the wide-ranging aspects of effective communication skills.

It is known that only 30% concerns the actual words; 20% is related to this in terms of intonation, etc., whereas the other 50% involves 'body language' (non-verbal communication). A person who stutters will often focus on the problem that they are having with interrupted speech. It is clear that by improving all aspects of communication, the person who stutters becomes more able to enter most situations with greater self-confidence. When a person enters a situation with a fear of speaking; an expectation of disaster; concentrating on 'tricks' and strategies in an attempt to avoid stuttering – it is likely to lead to failure. A vicious circle is the result:

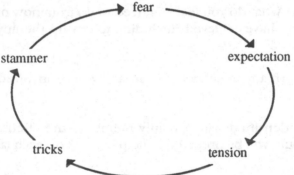

In contrast, a person who is able to enter situations with the knowledge that through observing the situation clearly, maintaining good eye-contact and facial expression, showing good listening skills through the use of acknowledgement and appropriate turntaking, he or she will feel more in control and more confident.

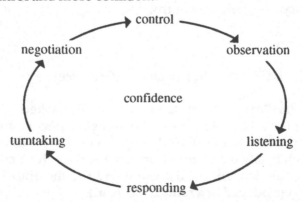

Greater control of speaking is a bonus!

This course has focused on:

1. *Speech production:* stuttering and fluency.
2. *Fluency control techniques:* the skill here is to be able to contrast the 'out of control' feeling of stuttering with the conscious and direct method of easy onsets, flowing the words and slowing the rate. The aim is to be able to alternate, as necessary, between spontaneous speech and 'technique'. The greatest problem is the degree of concentration involved; the only solution is practice:
   * By yourself, (preferably with a tape recorder).
   * In easy situations.
   * In gradually more difficult situations, try to set yourself assignments as we did on the course. (Note. REMEMBER TO ACKNOWLEDGE YOUR ATTEMPTS AS WELL AS SUCCESSES.)
3. *Observation skills:* to ensure that each situation is assessed in a valid and realistic way, this contributes to the following:
   Listening skills: to promote the skill of competing on, at least, equal terms with others. Effective communication is dependent on good listening.
   Praise and reinforcement: to establish the value of positive reinforcement to others, and perhaps more importantly to self reinforce. Confidence grows when a person is able to acknowledge his or her own success, however small. Negative thoughts set the scene for failure.
4. *Turntaking:* this focused on the skills required in conversations and requires good observation and listening.
5. *Problem-solving:* this technique develops the ability to find alternative solutions to problem. Remember the sequence:

* Generate as many ideas as possible.
* Discard the impossible, inadvisable, ineffective.
* Rank order the possible ideas.
* Try the first, or combination.
* If unsuccessful—try the next.

6. Negotiation: this skills is directly related to problem-solving—but at a higher level. It promotes assertion and reduces conflict. It is dependent on observation, listening, reinforcement, turntaking and problem solving. The outcome is mutual compromise and confidence.

A final thought

A problem that is kept as a deeply guarded secret; never discussed; never acknowledged—will not resolve by itself.

By attending this course you have taken a major step forward in confronting the problem. We all recognise and respect the courage that this has required.

Having overcome this hurdle, you have established the foundations for developing the skills of communication.

We look forward to seeing you on the 'follow-up' visits. In the meantime, please do not hesitate to contact us—we are here to support you.

References

ADAMS, G.R., SHEA, J. AND KACERGUIS, M.A. (1978) Development of psychosocial maturity: a review of selected effects of schooling. *Urban Education*, 13, 255–282.

ADAMS, G.R. (1983) Social competence during adolescence: social sensitivity, locus of control, empathy and peer popularity. *Journal of Youth and Adolescence*, 12 (3), 203–209.

ANDERSON, S. AND MESSICK, S. (1974) Social competency in young children. *Developmental Psychology*, 10, 282–293.

ANDREWS, G. AND HARRIS, M. (1964) The syndrome of stuttering. *Clinics in Developmental Medicine*, 17. London: Spastics Society Medical Information Unit in association with Heinemann Medical Books.

ANDREWS, G. AND CUTLER, J. (1974) Stuttering therapy: the relation between changes in symptom level and attitudes. *Journal of Speech and Hearing Disorders*, 39, 312–319.

ANDREWS, G., CRAIG, A., FEYER, A.M., HODDINOTT, S., HOWIE, P. AND NEILSON, M. (1983) Stuttering: a review of research findings and theories circa 1982. *Journal of Speech and Hearing Disorders*, 48, 226–246.

ARGYLE, M. (1982) The contribution of social interaction research to social skills training. In: Wine, J.W. and Syme, M.D. (eds). *Social Competence*. New York: Guildford Press.

BADDLEY, A.D. AND GATHERCOLE, S.E. (1993) *Working Memory and Language*. Hove: Lawrence Erlbaum Associates.

BADDLEY, A.D. AND HITCH, G.J. (1974) Working memory. In: Bower, G. (Ed.). *The Psychology of Learning and Motivation*. New York: Academic Press.

BELSKY, J., LERNER, R. AND SPANNIER, G. (1984) *The Child in the Family*. London: Addison-Wesley.

BERNSTEIN (1981) Are there constraints on childhood disfluency? *Journal of Fluency Disorders*, 6, 341–350.

BERNSTEIN RATNER, N. (in press) Language and stuttering. *Proceedings of the 1st World Congress on Fluency Disorders*, Munich, August 1994.

BERNSTEIN RATNER, N. AND SIH, C.C. (1987) Effects of gradual increases in sentence length and complexity on children's dysfluency. *Journal of Speech and Hearing Research*, 52, 278–287.

BLOODSTEIN, O. (1970) Stuttering and normal nonfluency—a continuity hypothesis. *British Journal of Disorders of Communication*, 5, 30–39.

BLOODSTEIN, O. (1987) *A Handbook on Stuttering* (4th edition). Chicago: National Easter Seal Society.

BLOTCKY, A.D. (1984) A framework for assessing the psychological functioning of adolescents. *Developmental and Behavioural Pediatrics*, 5, 74–77.

BOYSEN, A.E. AND CULLINAN, W.L. (1971) Object-naming latency in stuttering and nonstuttering children. *Journal of Speech and Hearing Research*, 14, 728–738.

CHANDLER, T.A., WOLD, F.M., COOK, B. AND DUGUVICE, B.A. (1980) Parental correlates of locus of control in fifth graders: an attempt at experimentation in the home. *Merrill-Palmer Quarterly*, 26, 183–195.

COLEMAN, J.C. AND HENDRY, L. (1990) *The Nature of Adolescence*. London: Routledge.

CONTURE, E.G. (1982) *Stuttering*. Englewood Cliffs, NJ: Prentice-Hall.

COOPER, E.B. AND RUSTIN, L. (1985) Clinician attitudes towards stuttering in the United States and Great Britain: a cross cultural study. *Journal of Fluency Disorders*, 10, 1–17.

CRAIG, A., FRANKLIN, J. AND ANDREWS, G. (1984) A scale to measure locus of control of behaviour. *British Journal of Medical Psychology*, 57, 173–180.

CRAIG, A. AND ANDREWS, G. (1985) The prediction and prevention of relapse in stuttering; the value of self control techniques and locus of control measures. *Behaviour Modification*, 9, 427–442.

DAMICO, J.S. (1985) Clinical discourse analysis: a functional approach to language assessment. In: Simon, C.S. (Ed.). *Assessment of Language-learning Disabled Students — Communication Skills and Classroom Success*. San Diego: College-Hill Press.

DANIELSON, J. AND SAMPSON, L. (1992) *Question the Information—Techniques for Classroom Listening*. East Moline, IL: Linguisystems.

DUNN, L.M., DUNN, L.M., WHETTON, C. AND PINTILLIE, D. (1982) *The British Picture Vocabulary Scales*. Windsor: NFER-Nelson.

EHREN, B.J. (1994) New directions in meeting the academic needs of adolescents with language learning disabilities. In: Wallach, G.P. and Butler, K.G. (eds). *Language Learning Disabilities in School-age Children and Adolescents—Some Principles and Applications*. New York: Macmillan College Publishing Company.

EPSTEIN, N., SCHLESINGER, S. AND DRYDEN, W. (1988) Concepts and methods of cognitive–behavioral family treatment. In: Epstein, N., Schlesinger, S. and Dryden, W. (eds). *Cognitive–Behavioural Therapy with Families*. New York: Brunner-Mazel.

ERIKSON, E.H. (1968) *Identity: Youth and Crisis*. New York: W.W. Norton.

FENWICK, E. AND SMITH, A. (1993) *Adolescence: The Survival Guide for Parents and Teenagers*. London: Dorling Kindersley.

GERMAN, D.J. (1990) *Test of Adolescent/Adult Word Finding*. Leicester: Taskmaster Ltd (UK Distributors).

GERMAN, D.J. (1993) *The Word Finding Intervention Program* (WFIP). Tucson, AZ: Communication Skill Builders.

GERMAN, D.J. (1994) Word finding difficulties in children and adolescents. In: Wallach, G.P. and Butler, K.G. (eds). *Language Learning Disabilities in School-age Children and Adolescents—Some Principles and Applications. New York: Macmillan College Publishing Company*.

GLASNER, P.J. AND ROSENTHAL, D. (1957) Parental diagnosis of stuttering in young children. *Journal of Speech and Hearing Disorders*, 22, 288–295.

GREENBERGER, E. AND SORENSON, A.B. (1974) Toward a concept of psychosocial maturity. *Journal of Youth and Adolescence*, 3, 329–358.

GREGORY, H. (1993) Closing summary, Oxford Dysfluency Conference, August 1994.

GUITAR, B. AND BASS, C. (1978) Stuttering therapy: the relation between attitude change and long term outcome. *Journal of Speech and Hearing Disorders*, 43, 392–400.

HALEY, J. (1973) *Uncommon Therapy: The Psychiatric Techniques of Milton H.*

Erickson. New York: Newton.

HALEY, J. (1980) *Leaving Home: The Therapy of Disturbed Young People*. New York: McGraw-Hill.

HAMMILL, D.D., BROWN, V., LARSEN, S. AND WIEDERHOLT, J. (1994) *Test of Adolescent and Adult Language* (third edition). Leicester: Taskmaster Ltd (UK Distributors).

HARKAWAY, J.E. (ED.) *Eating Disorders*. Rockville, MA: Aspen.

HOWIE, P.M. (1981) Concordance for stuttering in monozygotic and dizygotic twin pairs. *Journal of Speech and Hearing Research*, 24, 317–321.

JACOBSON, E. (1938) *Progressive Relaxation*. Chicago: University of Chicago Press.

JOHNSON, D.W. AND JOHNSON, F.P. (1975) *Joining Together: Group Theory and Group Skills*. Englewood Cliffs, NJ: Prentice-Hall.

JOHNSON W., DARLEY, F. AND SPRIESTERSBACH, D.C. (1952) *Diagnostic Manual in Speech Correction*. New York: Harper & Row.

JOHNSON-LAIRD, P.N. (1983). *Mental Models*. Cambridge, MA: Harvard University Press.

KELLY, G.A. (1955) *The Psychology of Personal Constructs*. New York: Norton.

KIDD, K.K. (1977) A genetic perspective on stuttering. *Journal of Fluency Disorders*, 2, 259–269.

KIDD, K. (1984) Stuttering as a genetic disorder. In: Curlee, R.F. and Perkins, W.H. (eds). *Nature and Treatment of Stuttering, New Directions*. San Diego: College Hill Press.

KIDD, K.K., KIDD, J.R. AND RECORDS, M.A. (1978) The possible causes of the sex ratio in stuttering and its implications. *Journal of Fluency Disorders*, 3, 13–23.

KIFER, R., LEWIS, M., GREEN, D. AND PHILLIPS, E. (1974) Training predelinquent youths and their parents to negotiate conflict situations. *Journal of Applied Behavior Analysis*, 7, 357–364.

KLEIN, H. (1985) The assessment of some persistent language difficulties in the learning disabled. In: Snowling, M.J. (Ed.) *Children's Written Language Difficulties*. London: Routledge.

KLEIN, H., CONSTABLE, A., GOULANDRIS, N., STACKHOUSE, J. AND TARPLEE, C. (1994) CELF–R^{UK}: Clinical Evaluation of language formation—Revised UK version. London: Psychological Corporation Ltd.

KLINE, M.L. AND STARKWEATHER, C.W. (1979) Receptive and expressive language performance in young stutterers. *ASHA*, 21, 797 (abstract).

LAHEY, M. AND BLOOM, L. (1994) Variability and language learning disabilities. In: Wallach, G.P. and Butler, K.G. (eds). *Language Learning Disabilities in School-age Children and Adolescents—Some Principles and Applications*. New York: Macmillan College Publishing Company.

LAZZARI, A.M. AND MYERS PETERS, P. (1987) *Handbook of Exercises for Language Processing*. (HELP) series. East Moline, IL: Linguisystems.

LEES, R.M. (in press) Of what value is a measure of the stutterer's fluency? *Folia Phonatrica*.

LEFCOURT, H.M. (1966) Locus of control—current trends. *Psychological Bulletin*, 65, 106–220.

LEFCOURT, H.M. (1976) *Locus of Control Current Trends: Theory and Research*. New York: Prentice-Hall.

LEFCOURT, H.M. (1982) *Current Trends in Theory and Research*. New York.

LERNER, R.M. (1985) Adolescent maturational changes and psychosocial development; a dynamic interactional perspective. *Journal of Youth and Adolescence*, 14, 355–372.

LIFSCHITZ, M. (1973) Internal–external locus of control dimension as a function of age and the socialisation milieu. *Child Development*, 44, 538–546.

LIVING AND LEARNING (1983) *Reading for Comprehension*. Cambridge: Learning Development Aids.

MALLARD, A.R. (1991) Using families to help the school age stutterer: a case study. In: Rustin, L. (Ed.). *Parents, Families and the Stuttering Child*. London: Whurr.

MCCONKEY, R. (1985) *Working With Parents*. London: Croom Helm.

MCGOLDRICK, M. AND GERSON, R. (1985) *Genograms in Family Assessment*. New York: W.W. Norton & Co.

MINUCHIN, S. (1974) *Families and Family Therapy*. Boston, MA: Harvard University Press.

MITCHELL, L. (1988) *Simple Relaxation: The Physiological Method for Easing Tension*. London: John Murray.

MOON, C. (1990) Miscue made simple. *Child Education*, November issue, 42–43.

MULHALL, D. (1977) *Personal Questionnaire Rapid Sealing Technique*. Windsor: NFER-Nelson.

MURRAY, H.L. AND REED C.G. (1977) Language abilities of preschool stuttering children. *Journal of Fluency Disorders*, 2, 171–176.

NEAVES, A.I. (1970) To establish a basis for prognosis in stammering. *British Journal of Disorders of Communication*, 5, 46–58.

NICHOLS, K.A. (1974) Severe social anxiety. *British Journal of Medical Psychology*, 47, 301–306.

NOWICKI, S., JNR AND STRICKLAND, B.R. (1973) A locus of control scale for children. *Journal of Consulting and Clinical Psychology*, 40 (1), 148–154.

NIPPOLD, M.A. (1990) Concomitant speech and language disorders in stuttering children: a critique of the literature. *Journal of Speech and Hearing Disorders*, 55, 51–60.

OKASHA, A., BISHRY, Z., KAMEL, M. AND HASSAN, A.H. (1974) Psychosocial study of stammering in Egyptian children. *British Journal of Psychiatry*, 124, 531–533.

OSTER, G.D., CARO, J.E., EAGEN, D.R. AND LILLO, M.A. (1988) *Assessing Adolescents*. London: Pergamon Press.

PERKINS, D. (1947) An item by item compilation and comparison of the scores of 75 young adult stutterers on the *California Test of Personality*, Speech Monograph, 14, 211.

PERKINS, W.H. (1979) From psychoanalysis to discoordination. In: Gregory, H.H. (Ed.). *Controversies About Stuttering Therapy*. Baltimore: University Park Press.

PERKINS, W.H. (1992) *Stuttering Prevented*. San Diego: Singular Publishing.

PETERS, T.J. AND GUITAR, B. (1991) *Stuttering: An Integrated Approach to Its Nature and Treatment*. Baltimore: Williams & Wilkins.

PRIESTLY, P., MCGUIRE, J., FLEGG, D., HEMSLEY, V. AND WELHAM, D. (1978) *Social Skills and Personal Problem Solving*. London: Tavistock.

PRINS, D. (1972) Personality, Stuttering severity, and age. *Journal of Speech and Hearing Research*, 15, 148–154.

PRINS, D. AND INGHAM, R.J. (1983) *Treatment of Stuttering in Early Childhood: Methods and Issues*. San Diego: College Hill Press.

QUINN, P.T. AND ANDREWS, G. (1977) Neurological stuttering—a clinical entity? *Journal of Neurology, Neurosurgery and Psychiatry*, 40, 699–701.

ROTTER, J.B. (1966) Generalized expectancies for internal versus external control of reinforcement. *Psychological Monographs*, 80, 1–28.

RUBIN, K.H. AND ROSS, H.S. (1982) Introduction: some reflections on the state of the art: the study of peer relationships and social skills. In: Rubin, K.H. and Ross, H.S. (eds). *Peer Relationships and Social Skills in Childhood*. New York: Springer.

RUSTIN, L. (1984) Intensive treatment models for adolescent stuttering: a comparison of social skills training and speech fluency techniques. Unpublished M.Phil. Thesis, Leicester Polytechnic.

RUSTIN, L. (1987) *Assessment and Therapy Programme for Disfluent Children*. Windsor: NFER-Nelson.

RUSTIN, L. (1991) *Parents, Families, and the Stuttering Child*. London: Whurr.

RUSTIN, L. AND COOK, F. (1983) Intervention procedures for the disfluent child. In: Dalton, P. (Ed.). *Approaches to the Treatment of Stuttering*. London: Croom Helm.

RUSTIN, L. AND COOK, F. (1995) Parental involvement in the treatment of stuttering. *Language, Speech and Hearing*.

RUSTIN, L. AND KUHR, A. (1989) *Social Skills and the Speech Impaired*. London: Whurr.

RUSTIN, L. AND PURSER, H. (1983) Intensive treatment models for adolescent stuttering: social skills versus speech techniques. Proceedings of the XIX Congress of the IALP, Edinburgh.

SCOTT, C.M. (1994) A discourse continuum for school-age students: impact of modality and genre. In: Wallach, G.P. and Butler, K.G. (eds). *Language Learning Disabilities in School-age Children and Adolescents—Some Principles and Applications*. New York: Macmillan College Publishing Company.

SEIDER, R.A., GLADSTEIN, K.L. AND KIDD, K.K. (1982) Language onset and concomitant speech and language problems in subgroups of stutterers and their siblings. *Journal of Speech and Hearing Research*, 25, 482–486.

SEMEL, E., WIIG, E.H., SECORD, W. (1987) *Clinical Evaluation of Language Fundamentals —Revised*. London: The Psychological Corporation.

SEMEL, E., WIIG, E.H., SECORD, W. (1989) *Clinical Evaluation of Language Fundamentals —Revised Screening Test*. London: The Psychological Corporation.

SHEEHAN, J.G. (1970) *Stuttering: Research and Therapy*. New York: Harper & Row.

SHEEHAN, J.G. (1975) Conflict theory and avoidance-reduction therapy. In: Eisenson, J. (Ed.). *Stuttering: A Second Symposium*. New York: Harper & Row.

SMITH, P. AND TOMPKINS, G. (1988) A new strategy for content area readers. *Journal of Reading*, 32, 46–53.

SPENCE, A. AND SPENCE, S. (1980) Cognitive changes associated with social skills training. *Behavioural Research and Therapy*, 18, 265–272.

STACKHOUSE, J. AND WELLS, B. (1993) Psycholinguistic assessment of developmental speech disorders. *European Journal of Disorders of Communication*, 27, 35–54.

STARKWEATHER, C.W. (1987) *Fluency and Stuttering*. Englewood Cliffs: Prentice-Hall.

STARKWEATHER, C.W. (1993) Issues of efficacy of treatment for fluency disorders. *Journal of Fluency Disorders*, 18, 151–168.

TROWER, P., BRYANT, B. AND ARGYLE, M. (1978) *Social Skills and Mental Health*. London: Methuen.

VAN RIPER, C. (1982) *The Nature of Stuttering* (second edition). Englewood Cliffs: Prentice-Hall.

WALL, M.J. (1977) The location of stuttering in the spontaneous speech of young child stutterers. Ph.D. dissertation. New York: City University of New York.

WALL, M.J. (1980) A comparison of syntax in young stutterers and nonstutterers. *Journal of Fluency Disorders*, 5, 345–352.

WATZLAWICK, P. (1984) *The Invented Reality*. New York: Norton.

WEINS, A.N. AND MATARAZZO, J.D. (1983) Diagnostic interviewing. In: Hersen, M., Kazdin, A.E. and Bellack, A.S. (eds). *The Clinical Psychology Handbook*. New York: Pergamon

WESTBY, C.E. (1974) Language performance in stuttering and nonstuttering children. *Journal of Communication Disorders*, 12, 133–145.

WILLIAMS, D.E., MELROSE, B.M. AND WOODS, C.L. (1969). The relationship between stuttering and academic achievement in children. *Journal of Communication Disorders*, 2, 87–98.

WINGATE, M.E. (1962) Personality need of stutters. *LOGOS*, 5, 35–37.

WINGATE, M.E. (1976) *Stuttering Theory and Treatment*, New York: Invington.

WOOLF, G. (1967) The assessment of stuttering as struggle, avoidance and expectancy. *British Journal of Disorders of Communication*, 2, 158–171.

WRIGHT, J.D. AND PEARL, L. (1986) Knowledge and experience of young people of drug abuse 1969–84. *British Medical Journal*, 292, 179–182.

YAIRI, E. (1983) The onset of stuttering in two- and three-year-old children: a preliminary report. *Journal of Speech and Hearing Disorders*, 48, 171–178.

YAIRI, E. (1993) Epidemiologic and other considerations in treatment efficacy research with preschool-age children who stutter. *Journal of Fluency Disorders*, 18 (2 and 3).

ZARB, J.M. (1992) *Cognitive Behavioural Assessment and Therapy with Adolescents*. New York: Brunner-Mazel.

Index

adolescence
  communication skills approach
    57–70
  depression 23
  developmental psychology 7–8
  drugs, solvents, alcohol 24, 148
  eating disorders 22, 147
  empathy 30, 36
  family 22–3
  Lifespan Developmental Psychology
    7–8
  locus of control 9, 12–13, 30–2, 41
  parental perceptions 99, 181–2
  personality growth 7
  physical changes 7
  self-image 1, 7, 9, 11, 21, 24, 29, 36
  sexual behaviour 21
  social communication skills 10–11,
    13
  social competency 30, 31
  social knowledge 30
  social relationships 147
  social roles 7
  speech and language impairment
    8–13
  stuttering 2, 8–13
adolescent(s)
  as active agent 8
  as agent, shaper and selector 8
  assessment of - summarising 17, 27
  case history, interviewing - opening,
    closing 17–18, 26–7
  depression 46
  parents, teachers, siblings 7
  planning intervention therapy with
    school 56, 123–4

  as processor 8
  as stimulus 8
aetiology
  capacities and demands theory 4–5,
    8–9
  communicative failure and anticipa-
    tory struggle 57
  constitutional factors 3–4
    interaction with
    developmental/environmental
    factors 3
  developmental factors
    cognitive 4
    physical 4
    social and emotional 4
    speech and language 4
  environmental factors
    family 4, 5
    heredity 3, 46, 53, 54
    life events 4
    parents 4–5
    peers 4
    perceptions of others 4
    school 4
    society 5
    teachers 4
anticipation
  of failure 41, 50
  of stuttering 40, 53
articulation disorders in adolescents
    who stutter 127
assertion continuum 68, 94–5
assertive behaviour 36
assertive skills 9
assessment
  academic achievement 21

adolescents, of adolescents who stut-
    ter 15–18
attitude questionnaires 29
audiotape recording 18
of avoidance strategies 29, 33–4, 35
behavioural factors 39, 42, 47, 51, 54
belief systems 41
case history form 38
cognitive behaviour 19
cognitive-emotional factors 35–6,
    38–9, 41–2, 47, 54
commencing an 17–18, 26–7
core stuttering behaviour 19
and diagnosis 18–25
empathy 36
environmental factors 39–40, 42, 47,
    51, 54–5
family 16, 26–8, 110
feedback from 28
feelings and attitudes 18, 19, 21,
    28–9
fluency 18–19, 74, 133–5, 143
formal 25, 29, 130–1
guidelines for 15–36
informal 16–25
linguistic skills 25–6, 130–1
locus of control 30–2, 35, 74
non-verbal IQ 34–5
parental attitudes, parental interview
    26–8
parents 23
phonological development in stutter-
    ers 3, 4
physiological factors 38–9, 41, 46–7,
    51, 53
PQRST 29, 36, 48, 74, 103
principles of 15
range of 18–25
rate of speech 34
rationale for 15–16
secondary stuttering behaviours 6
self-image 29, 36
social background 22–4
social communication skills 30, 75
social knowledge 30
speech and language delay 3, 4
of stuttering behaviour 33, 153
summarising the findings of 17, 27,
    43
terminating an 26, 27
treatment planning 37, 38

verbal IQ 33–4
videotape recording 18
attitudes
    of adolescents 7
    of adolescents who stutter 2, 9, 29,
        53, 145
    assessment of 18, 19, 21, 28–9
    client questionnaires on 29
    clinicians 2
    empathy 30, 58
    of family 4
    investigating 25
    and locus of control 12–13, 61–2
    of parents 11, 50, 111–12
    of peers 24, 125, 147
    of society 15
    stuttering modification therapy and
        44, 49, 52, 55
    of teachers 20, 54
avoidance behaviours
    of adolescents who stutter 6, 35, 50,
        53, 133
    identifying 33–4, 46
    self-assessment of 29

behaviour
    of adolescents 39
    anti-social 155
    assertive 36
    avoidance 6, 29, 33–4, 35, 46, 50, 53,
        133
    cognitive and behaviour therapy 58,
        59
    core 5–6
    discipline and 23–4
    problems 25
    secondary 6
    stuttering 19
body language
    and proximity 71
    and social competence 85
    and social skills 184

capacities and demands theory 128–9
    constitutional factors and 3
    developmental factors and 4–5
    environmental factors and 4–5
    Sheehan's contributions to 11
    Starkweather's view of 4–5, 128
capacity for fluency 4–5, 8–9

case history
    adolescents 19–25
    approach to 16
    clinician's role in 16
    elements of 19–25
    families 26–8
    importance of 16
    parents 26–8
    range of 18–25
    taking of 19–28
case studies of stuttering in adolescence
    central auditory processing 135–8
    cognitions and behavioural change
        in adolescents 40–1, 44–6, 49–50,
        52–4, 111–12, 115, 117, 120, 122,
        124, 125
        in parents 40, 41, 45, 46, 50, 53,
        111–12, 115, 117, 122
        in teachers 54, 124
    cognitive
        and behavioural therapy 42, 47,
        51, 54
        restructuring 17
        therapy for adolescents 40–56
    communication skills approach
        listening 67
        negotiation 68
        and observation 66–7
        parents' involvement 68–9
        praise and reinforcement 67–8
        problem-solving 68, 120
        turntaking 67
checklist
    communication skills 75, 118, 120,
    160–1
    self-rating 161
communication failure 57
    constitutional factors and 3–4
    developmental factors and 4–5
    environmental factors and 4–5
constitutional factors
    capacities and demands theory and 3
    communication failure and 3
    stuttering and 1, 3–4
core behaviours
    of adolescents who stutter 6
    of normal dysfluency 6
    of stuttering 5–6

demands for fluency 4
developmental factors

capacities and demands theory and
    4–5
    cognitive development 4
    physical development 4
    social and emotional development 4
    speech and language development 4
    in stuttering behaviour 1, 4–5
developmental history 158
development of stuttering 3, 4, 5
    and severity 6
diagnosis
    and assessment 18–25
    diagnostic interviewing 18–25
    framework for 32–6, 38–40
    and treatment planning 37–8
    use of case history grid for 38
dysfluency
    and the adolescent 19, 29, 31
    assessment of 74
    categories of 6
    characteristics of 129
    core behaviours of 5–6
    feelings and attitudes about 19, 29,
    31
    and group therapy 74, 82
    and individual therapy 19, 26
    secondary behaviours of 6
    summary of 26, 27, 151
    types of 6, 74

environmental factors
    and the adolescent 8, 39–40
    and behavioural factors 39
    and cognitive emotional factors 39
    and constitutional factors 1, 3
    and developmental factors 1, 4–5
    and their effect upon stuttering
        behaviour 4–5, 11, 39–40
    family 3, 5, 68, 110–12, 113
    heredity 3, 151
    parents 4–5, 11–12, 68–9, 110–12,
    113–16
    peers 124–6
    perceptions of stress 35
    schools 122–3
    siblings 111
    society 15
    teachers 123–4
eye-contact 34, 49–50, 66, 85, 89, 184

facial expression 35, 184

families
  and the adolescent 2, 22–3, 42,
    147–8, 154
  assessment 22–3, 26, 155–7
  case history taking and 16, 22–3, 26
  counselling 110–11
  heredity 3, 46
  and homework tasks 119
  importance of 4, 22–3, 26, 42
  influence of 2, 4, 5, 47
  involvement in therapy 2, 69, 105,
    110–11, 113, 117, 120–1
  partnership with 69, 120–1
  perceptions of stuttering 4
  training 105
family studies 155–7, 183
fear
  of failure 41, 50
  of situations 46, 50
  of stuttering 179
feelings
  assessment of adolescents 18, 19, 21,
    28–9
  client questionnaires on - for adoles-
    cents 29
  stuttering modification therapy and
    44, 49, 52, 55
fluency
  breath control 63
  capacity for 4–5, 8–9
  controlled 60–4, 185
  demands for 4
  dimensions of 18–19, 74, 133–5, 143
  easy onsets 63, 84
  environmental influences on 4
  feasibility of 60
  flow of speech 63, 84
  improving control of 60–4
  maintenance of 10, 13, 30
  and normal dysfluency 60, 62, 82
  parents' response to 46, 60
  rate 63
  rate control 63
  soft contacts 63–4
  speech naturalness and 62–3, 64
  transfer of 10, 103
fluency goals
  of communication skills approach 60
  of fluency-shaping therapy 60
  of integrated approach 60
  of stuttering modification therapy 60

fluency-shaping therapy
  comparison with stuttering 60
  modification 25
foundation skills
  family studies of 155–7, 183
  heredity 3, 151
  listening 67
  observation 66–7
  praise and reinforcement 67–8
  social communication skills 65–6

homework assignments/tasks 82, 84, 87,
    93
integrated approach
  client's understanding of own
    stuttering behaviour 66
  establishing long-term fluency
    goals 91
  fluency goals 91, 97
  measuring outcomes 28
  monitoring progress 76–7
  parents' role in therapy 97
  self-evaluation 97
  transfer of fluency 76–7

intelligence, assessment of 3
interaction skills
  empathy 30, 51
  listening 67
  locus of control 9, 12–13, 30–2
  meta-perception 66
  observation 30, 34, 48, 66–7
  praise and reinforcement 67–8
  problem-solving, negotiation 48, 68
  social competency 10–11
  social knowledge 30
  turntaking 35, 67
interview
  and the adolescent 17–18, 144–50
  clinical 16–18
  clinician's role 25, 37–8
  closing 26, 27, 37–8
  conducting 17, 19–25, 27
  diagnostic 18–25
  family/parental 16, 26–8, 153–9
  introducing 17–18, 26–7
  opening 17–18, 26–7
  summarising 17, 27, 38

language, development of 1, 3, 4, 127,
    135–6

language disorders
    assessment of in adolescents 129–31
    stuttering and 127–8
listening
    locus of control
        and the adolescent 34–5
        empathy 177
        and maintenance of fluency 185
        peer relationships 90
        problem-solving 68
        social competence 67
        social knowledge 87–9, 184

modelling fluent speech 128
Modified Erickson Scale of communication attitudes 29, 35, 74

non-verbal behaviour 67
non-verbal communication 67

observation 30, 34, 66–7, 85, 118–19, 177, 185
onset of stuttering 1, 5, 41, 151
outcome measures 32–6
    efficacy 33
    and evaluation 32–3
    as measures of 33, 162–6

parents
    and adolescents 11–12, 23–4, 41–2, 181–2
    assessment of interaction with adolescents 23, 110, 148, 157
    attitudes 11–12, 23–4, 111–12
    child-rearing styles 12–13, 111, 112–13, 114
    conflict 23, 42, 116
    and contingency contracting 121–2
    discipline regimes 23–4, 112, 148–9, 157
    expectations 4, 42, 47, 51
    interaction checklist 118, 120
    interviews 16, 17, 153–9
    involvement in therapy 11, 12, 43–4, 68–9, 72, 95–7, 98–101, 113–16
    language 5
    marital therapy/counselling 43, 52
    and negotiation skills training 121
    as partners 68–9
    reactions to fluency 4

reactions to stuttering 11, 50, 111–12
    speech of 5, 46, 50, 55
    video feedback 112, 115
peers
    and adolescence 22, 69, 154
    alcohol 24
    bullying 125
    drugs 24
    importance of 69
    influence of 24
    involvement of in therapy 70
    range of 50, 147
    same sex and opposite sex 147
    social network 42, 47, 124–5
    social skills 54
    teasing 125, 147
positive feedback 56
praise and reinforcement 67–8, 93–4, 118–19, 178, 185
problem-solving
    communication skills approach and 68, 185
    and locus of control 31, 112
    and negotiation skills 121, 185
    as part of therapy 36, 95, 97, 119–21

rate of speech 5, 9, 41, 47
    assessment of 19, 34
rating scales
    inter-rater reliability and outcome measures 33
    self-rating 29, 34, 35, 36, 95, 161
recovery
    in females 5
    remission 5, 8–9
    spontaneous 1, 5
reinforcement
    praise and 93–4, 118–19, 178, 185
    skills 67–8
relaxation
    Jacobson 65
    Mitchell 65
    training 65, 86, 89, 90
role play 66, 93
role rehearsal 52

scale, self-rating 29, 34, 35, 36, 95, 161
school
    adolescents and 20–2, 122–3, 145–6, 155
    discipline at 20

liaison with 55, 56, 123–4
peer pressure and 24
performance at 21, 146
problems in 123–4, 146
programmes in 123–4
teachers 20, 123–4
working with 55, 56, 69–70, 123–4
self-image 1, 7, 9, 11, 21, 24, 29, 36, 175
self-rating scales 29, 34, 35, 36, 95, 161
self-worth 67–8
sensory motor coordination 8
sensory motor processing 3, 8
sex ratio 5–6, 151
    heredity and 3
sexual behaviour
    and adolescence 21
    case history 21, 42
    identification of 155
    questioning about 21, 146–7
situational avoidance by adolescents
        who stutter 35, 46, 50
situation fears 46, 50
social adjustment 10
social communication skills 30, 42, 48,
        57–8, 75
social competency
    empathy 30
    locus of control 30, 31
    social knowledge 30
social development 30
social interaction 9, 22, 42, 47, 57–8, 147
social psychology 26
social relationships
    and adolescence 22
    with authority figures 154
    within the family 154
    with peers 22, 124
    within school 22, 147
social skills
    categories of 65, 66–8
    cognitive behaviour therapy 66
    elements of 13, 30, 54, 160–1
    hierarchy of 30, 71
    generalisation of 10–11
    teaching 65, 84–5, 138
    training
        effectiveness of 53
        structure of therapy 66–8
soft contacts 63–4
speech
    of adolescents 25, 153

assessment of 19–20
development of 1
dysfluency and motor control of 8
effort of 62
parents' expectations for 4, 42
rate of 9, 19, 34, 63, 151
stresses on 11–12
of stutterer's parents 5
taperecording of 18, 62
videorecording of 18, 62
stutterer
    adolescent 8–13
    capacities of 4–5
    demands upon 4–5
    intelligence of 3
    parents of 4, 11–12
    school performance of 21
    sensory motor coordination of 3
    speech and language development of
        1, 3
stuttering
    adaptiveness of 47, 51
    and adolescence 8–13
    aetiology of 2–3, 5, 151
    anticipation of 40, 53
    articulation disorders and 127
    assessment of 33, 145
    case studies of 40–1, 44–6, 49–50,
        52–4
    causes of 2–3, 5
    cerebral dominance and 3
    cognitive development and 3
    components of 132–3
    consistency of 46
    core behaviours of 5–6
    definition of 60–1
    developmental 3, 4
    and the effect of constitutional devel-
        opmental factors 3–5
    effect of treatment on 44, 49, 52,
        55–6
    environmental factors 4–5
    epidemiology of 128–9, 151
    feelings and attitudes about 18, 19,
        21, 28–9, 53
    heritability of 3, 46, 151
    incidence of 3, 46, 151
    incidence of 3, 5
    IQ and
        non-verbal IQ 3
        verbal IQ 3

language disorders 129–30
linguistic development and 1,3, 4,
    135–6
linguistic factors and 127–9, 151
modification of 25, 150
onset of 1, 5, 41, 151
open discussion of 11
parental attitudes to words 111–12,
    122
percentage words affected by 19, 49,
    53
phonological development and 134
predisposing and precipitating
    factors in 3–5
prevalence of 5
psychological factors 3, 5
secondary behaviours of 6
sensory motor processing and 8
sex ratio of 5–6, 151
speech and language delay and 3, 5
spontaneous recovery from 1, 5
'subclinical' features of 3, 64
variability of 19
voice onset and 3, 127, 135–6
stuttering severity index for adolescents
    143
suicide attempts 45, 46, 47, 113

taperecording 18, 62
teachers
    and adolescents who stutter 20, 54,
        56, 123–4, 146

counselling of 124
discipline 20
influence of 20
involvement of 55, 56, 123–4, 139
as partners in training programme
    55, 56, 69–70, 123–4
relationships between adolescents
    and 20, 54
working with clinicians 55, 123–4
teasing
    coping with 125, 147
    elimination of 125
    by peers 125, 147
    problem-solving of 147
    by teachers 21
treatment
    of adolescents who stutter 43–4,
        48–9, 51–2, 55–6
    assessment of 87
    clinician's belief about 2
    diagnosis for 38, 43–4
    effect of 44, 49, 52, 55–6
    efficacy of 62
    evaluation of 87
    goals of 58–9
    maintenance procedures and 58
    outcome measures and 32–3
    planning for 38–40
    range of 59–70
    self-reinforcement as part of 58
    transfer of fluency within 58

9 781897 635605